CREATING HEALTH
The Psychophysiological Connection

CREATING HEALTH

The Psychophysiological Connection

Deepak Chopra, M.D., F.A.C.P.

VANTAGE PRESS
New York / Washington / Atlanta
Los Angeles / Chicago

The author is grateful to Carol Sparling, CMT, for the typing of this manuscript.

FIRST EDITION

Published by Vantage Press, Inc.
516 West 34th Street, New York, New York 10001

Manufactured in the United States of America
ISBN: 0-533-06007-9

Library of Congress Catalog Card No.: 83-91014

To Maharishi Mahesh Yogi, whose extraordinary insight into the
nature of intelligence restructured my reality

Contents

Part I
Health and Disease

Part II
Laying the Foundation

Part III
Strategies for Healthier and Happier Living

Part IV
Toward a Higher Reality—Meditation and Metamorphosis

CREATING HEALTH
The Psychophysiological Connection

Part I
Health and Disease

Chapter One

Introduction: How To Be Perfectly Healthy and Remain Ever-Youthful

The World Health Organization has defined health not merely as the absence of disease or infirmity, but as a state of perfect physical, mental, and social well-being. To this may be added spiritual well-being, a state where the individual feels in every moment of living a joy and zest for living, a sense of fulfillment, and a sense of harmony with the universe around him. It would be a state where the individual feels ever-youthful, ever-buoyant, and ever-happy. Such a state is not only desirable, but quite possible. It is not only quite possible, it is easy to attain. This book intends to show you how you may attain perfect health and how you may remain ever-youthful.

Chapter Two

Ill Health

Any discussion of perfect health must also include a few words about ill health. Below is a list of some of the more common problems encountered in everyday clinical practice. In the next few chapters, I will deal specifically with each of these problems. I will tell you how the medical community deals with them (the conventional approach, with which I agree sometimes), and will tell you my approach (nonconventional at times, and I believe sometimes more effective).

After I have dealt with the common problems, I will devote the rest of the book to the perfection of health and to the maintenance of everlasting youth. In the end I will build a case for the practice of a mental technique that makes all this possible. It is up to the reader to decide for himself whether the technique works or not. He cannot decide this without trying it. So, if you are one of those people who is merely going to read this book without doing anything about it, then you are wasting your time. On the other hand, if you plan to at least try the suggestions, then read on—you have perfect health and everlasting youth to look forward to.

But first the common problems, and what the conventional and nonconventional thinking is about them. Here is a list of what I see every day in my office:

1. People with hypertension and cardiovascular disease and cerebro-vascular disease (high blood pressure, heart attack, and stroke).

2. People with cancer.
3. People with musculoskeletal problems, muscle aches and pains, arthritis, and backache.
4. People with anxieties and depression, sleep disorders, and other psychiatric disorders.
5. People with problems related to cigarette smoking, alcohol consumption, and drug abuse.
6. People with weight problems, either too much or too little (usually too much). They complain, "I don't eat a thing, but I can't lose any weight."
7. People with fatigue for which no medical cause can be determined. These people complain, "Why am I so tired all the time?"
8. People with sexual problems.
9. People with problems related to accidents, automobile accidents and other accidents.
10. People with glandular problems.
11. People with gastrointestinal (digestive) problems.
12. People with problems related to infection.

In the next few chapters, I will deal with most of these problems, devoting greater time and detail to some of the more common ones.

Chapter Three

High Blood Pressure, Heart Attack, and Stroke

Hypertension, or high blood pressure, is a very common disorder and afflicts a very high percentage of the population. If you are thirty or older, you have at least a one-in-five chance of being hypertensive. What exactly is high blood pressure? The blood pressure is simply the pressure applied by the blood to the walls of the blood vessels. It is usually recorded in millimeters of mercury by an instrument called a sphygmomanometer. The pressure recorded at the time the heart is contracting is called the systolic pressure and should normally be less than 140 millimeters of mercury, and the pressure recorded at the time the heart is relaxing is called the diastolic pressure and should normally be less than 90 millimeters of mercury. In other words, normal blood pressure is less than 140/90. When blood pressure increases to over 140/90, we call it hypertension. Blood pressure increases normally with aging.

Hypertension is harmful and must be treated because it causes damage to vital organs, including the heart, the kidneys, and the brain. Untreated, it leads to heart failure, stroke, and kidney failure, and consequently to a reduced life span. What is the cause of high blood pressure? In the vast majority of patients, scientists have been unable to find a specific cause for high blood pressure. Thus, in more than 90 percent of people with hypertension, no clear reason for the elevated blood pressure can be given.

However, a number of interesting observations have been made. There is evidence that abnormal psychological stimuli may play a role in the genesis of hypertension. Experimentally chronically stressed animals can become hypertensive; psychological stress is frequently seen in patients with hypertension. Moreover, sedatives and tranquilizers have been used successfully in the treatment of hypertension. Therefore, most physicians associate "stress," particularly psychological stress (a non-tangible/tangible), with hypertension. We will deal later with some of the personality factors most frequently seen in stressed people.

Another factor implicated in the causation of high blood pressure is increased salt intake. People, as well as animals, can be made hypertensive if given a high intake of salt in their diet. (A full chapter on the role of diet and the causation of various disease processes is included later in the book.)

Recently a great deal of interest has developed in the role of hormones in hypertension. Hormones are certain chemicals produced by glandular structures in various parts of the body that have an effect on other parts of the body distant from the site of production of the hormones. In other words, hormones are chemical messengers. Hormones that may be altered in hypertension include cortisol, adrenaline, aldosterone, and renin. It is really not important to know the names. The important fact is that the concentration of certain chemicals is altered in the blood of the person with hypertension. Hypertension attributed to "stress" is felt to be mediated via hormones. It is felt that emotions such as fear, anxiety, hostility, and anger cause an alteration in certain chemicals in the brain. These chemicals, or neurotransmitters, as they are called, can in turn influence the secretion of hormones, such as ACTH from the pituitary. These in turn stimulate the adrenal glands (structures above the kidneys) which then release hormones such as cortisol and adrenaline into the blood, causing a rise in blood pressure. This is only one example of a phenomenon that is being increasingly recognized as a mechanism in the genesis of a disease process. The phenomenon, of course, is the translation of an emotion or thought into a chemical message, which in turn stimulates a distant organ.

Most of the effects studied have been for the elucidation of disease-producing mechanisms (since the consciousness of scientists and physicians is so disease-oriented). It is logical, therefore, that the opposite

7

kind of emotion should have a life-supporting and healthy influence on the body. In the foreseeable future, biologists will be studying the alteration in brain neurotransmitters that occurs with the introduction of such positive thoughts as love, compassion, peace, courage, faith. A very important recent observation has been that hormones formerly thought to be present in the blood stream *only* have also been discovered in significant concentration in brain tissue itself. Renin, a hormone secreted by the kidney and implicated in the organ damage that occurs in hypertension, is also found in brain tissue. Moreover, it in turn is influenced by the concentration of other hormones—such as somatostatin—which are present in the brain. Hormones are in turn influenced by alterations in neurotransmitter content. Neurotransmitters (also called biogenic amines) are just chemicals. The common ones are dopamine, serotinin, epinephrine, and norepinephrine.

It is only a matter of time before biologists will be able to demonstrate and identify the change in the concentration of various hormones and chemicals in the brain and in the body which occurs when a person changes his thought patterns. In a later chapter, I intend to explore the simple and elegant technologies that may be utilized to alter these thought patterns and emotions in a favorable direction so that body physiology may in turn be favorably affected.

CURRENT APPROACHES TO THE TREATMENT OF HYPERTENSION—AND THEIR LIMITATIONS

Drugs

Most physicians use various kinds of drugs to treat hypertension. The reason for this is two-fold. First, drugs are the quickest and easiest solution, both for the physician and the patient. In an economy which is geared to productivity, and at a time when the aim of the majority of physicians and people in general is to accomplish as much as possible with as little effort as possible, it is much easier for a physician to write a prescription than it is to sit down with a patient and go into all the reasons why he may be hypertensive, and the changes in life-style that may be necessary to bring his blood pressure down. Moreover, in the majority of cases, patients are not willing to change their life-styles and their dietary habits. It is so much easier to swallow a pill or a couple of pills, or, as we will see later, a lot of pills, and go about one's business.

The second reason drugs are the most popular modality for the treatment of hypertension and other diseases is that they are effective, and some of them are very effective. We live in a society which demands instant solutions to all problems. The quickest solution to a medical problem is to take a pill. The pharmaceutical industry and the scientific community have spent years and years of research and billions of dollars to develop some of the most effective pharmaceutical agents for the treatment of hypertension. So, if pills are so effective and so easy to take, what is the problem?

Problems and Limitations of Drug Therapy

1. Drugs are expensive. The costs of research for better products are, of course, passed on to the consumer. Some antihypertensive agents these days cost up to a dollar a pill, and a pill may have to be taken several times a day, sometimes for life.

2. All drugs, without exception, have side effects. There is no such thing as a perfect pill. Some of the common side effects associated with antihypertensive agents include fatigue, dryness of the mouth, blurred vision, disturbance of taste, sexual dysfunction (such as impotence), dizziness, lack of concentration and memory, emotional disturbance, increased irritability, sometimes severe depression, and damage to liver, kidney, and bone marrow. The list of possible side effects is lengthy. Many patients learn to live with the less serious and relatively "minor" side effects, such as a little fatigue and dryness of the mouth. However, there are a number of people who refuse to take a medicine because of its side effects, even though they realize that their hypertension is life-threatening and will shorten their life span. In fact, noncompliance is one of the major problems in the treatment of hypertension.

3. Drugs have to be taken for a lifetime, and a lot of people hate the idea of being dependent on something for the rest of their lives.

4. Drug tolerance, or tachyphylaxis. A frequently observed phenomenon in biology is that of tachyphylaxis, or drug tolerance. Drug

tolerance is said to occur when continued use of the drug ceases to be effective, or when larger doses are required to produce the same effect. Frequently in the treatment of hypertension a drug will no longer be effective after continued use, or larger doses will be required to produce the desired biological effect. With larger doses, of course, the likelihood of side effects will also increase.

So, we see there are several disadvantages in the treatment of hypertension by drugs.

What are some of the non-pharmacological approaches to the management of hypertension?

1. Diet

The lowering of salt intake in the diet is an effective means of lowering blood pressure if it is moderately elevated. Most physicians caution their patients against excessive salt intake. Since dietary habits are ingrained over a lifetime, patients find it very difficult to decrease their salt intake.

2. Mental Techniques

Several mental techniques have recently been popularized as being useful in the treatment of hypertension. These include: a) biofeedback; b) various relaxation techniques; c) visualization; and d) meditation.

Biofeedback. In this technique, the patient's arm is hooked up to a recording device which measures the patient's blood pressure. The patient can see on an instrument panel the fluctuations in blood pressure that occur spontaneously. He can then teach himself either to raise or lower the pressure by willing or desiring it to fluctuate in either direction. With the continuous feedback that he obtains from the instrument panel, he can train himself to effect any autonomic function, including the control of blood pressure. This is a fascinating example of the psycho-physiological connection where a desire can be translated into a physiological response. In practice, biofeedback, as it is currently available, is not a very effective means of controlling moderately severe hyper-

10

tension. However, the simple fact that a person can change his blood pressure by merely desiring to do so is in itself a fascinating and extremely important observation. It establishes once again the very important fact that a thought or desire can mediate a physiological response. Everybody is familiar with the fact that erotic or sexually arousing thoughts will result in a penile erection or lubrication of vaginal mucosa. Therefore, it should not be surprising that other thoughts or desires can result in other kinds of physiological response. The key thing to learn from these observations and studies on biofeedback is that we can change our blood pressure by changing our thought patterns.

Various Relaxation Techniques. These have also proved useful in the treatment of hypertension. Their use is limited at the moment to the treatment of very mild hypertension.

Visualization. This is another variation of relaxation where the individual visualizes, with his eyes closed, a calm and serene picture. The technique is useful in the treatment of mild hypertension.

Meditation. By far the most useful technique for lowering blood pressure is the technique known as Transcendental Meditation. It is also true that people who practice the TM technique on a regular basis do not develop hypertension. The topic of Transcendental Meditation is too important to discuss in this section, and I plan to devote an entire chapter to it later on in this book.

I have discussed in this section some of the causes, consequences, and current treatments of hypertension. It is apparent that most of the above-mentioned approaches are not ideal. What is the answer? Is there some means by which we can prevent hypertension before it occurs, and is there some means by which we can cure it once it occurs? I believe the key to this lies in our better understanding of ourselves. For that, of course, we will first have to define what we mean by the word "ourselves" or the word "self." Who or what is the "self"? This is the topic of another chapter and will be discussed in due course.

THE PROBLEM OF HEART DISEASE
AND HEART ATTACKS

Coronary artery disease is the number one killer in the United States and in the Western world. Coronary arteries are blood vessels that carry oxygen to the heart. When they become blocked, there is deprivation of oxygen to the heart muscle. This results in death of heart muscle or "myocardial infarction," the common medical terminology for heart attack. A severe heart attack, of course, results in death (usually within the first few hours of its onset). What are the common factors associated with heart attack? The following is a list of the common risk factors:

1. Obesity. Fat people are more likely than thin people to have heart attacks.
2. High blood pressure. We have already discussed this factor at length.
3. Stress. Psychological stress is considered to be a major factor in the genesis of coronary artery disease. A particular type of personality, defined as a Type A personality, is more prone to the development of coronary artery disease. Type A persons are aggressive, competitive, and tense. They are forever trying to "beat the deadline." Frequently hostility, fear, and anger are seen to be dominant emotions in Type A personalities.
4. Hypercholesterolemia, or increased cholesterol. Cholesterol is a fat, or lipid, in the blood and is more frequently elevated in the blood of persons with coronary artery disease. The biggest source of cholesterol is fat in our diet, particularly the animal fat contained in red meats.
5. Lack of physical exercise. Heart attacks more frequently occur in sedentary and physically inactive persons.
6. Smoking. In addition to cancer, smokers are much more likely to have heart attacks than non-smokers.
7. Other risk factors include being a member of the male sex, although this disparity is slowly disappearing as women acquire a lot of "male traits"; increasing age; and hereditary factors. (Patients with a strong family history of heart attack are more at risk.)

It should be obvious from an analysis of the above list that most of the factors are under our control. *We* can control obesity, high blood pressure, smoking, stress, physical activity, etc. Why is it that some of us are better at doing this and others are not so successful? The key, again, lies in a better understanding of ourselves, or the "self." As mentioned before, an attempt will be made later at defining and elucidating a better understanding of the "self."

STROKE

Stroke or shock occurs when one of the blood vessels going to the brain either becomes blocked or ruptures. Many of the same factors discussed earlier apply to the pathogenesis of stroke, although hypertension is a very frequent and predominant accompaniment of stroke.

Chapter Four

Cancer

Cancer is a term used to define an abnormal growth of cells in the body. The abnormal cells invade normal tissues and spread to other organs, causing dysfunction and finally death of these organs. It is estimated that one out of every four Americans will develop cancer during his lifetime. Although the exact cause of cancer at the molecular level is not yet defined, various environmental agents have been identified as causing cancer. The following is a list of various factors known to cause cancer:

Viruses. It is fairly well established that certain viruses can cause cancer. EB virus, which is usually the infectious agent in infectious mononucleosis, has, for example, been shown to cause Burkitt's lymphoma (cancer of the lymph glands). It has also been shown to cause nasopharyngeal cancer (cancer of the nose, and the cavity between mouth and esophagus). Obviously, all people who get mononucleosis do not develop cancer. In fact, only a very small proportion or even a miniscule proportion of the people exposed to this virus will develop cancer. Why is it that a virus will cause cancer in some people and not in others? The exact reason is not known. However, it seems that some people are more prone to develop a disease of any kind, including cancer.

A number of host factors are involved, including a condition called immunosuppression. Immunosuppression is a term used to denote decreased immunity or decreased ability to fight a disease, usually an infection or cancer. Immunosuppression, in turn, is a result of many factors, including poor nutrition. In some cases, immunosuppression is due to the production of the wrong kinds of antibodies, or antibodies that fail to distinguish between outside, harmful agents and the body's own cells. When this happens, that is, when the body's germ-fighting mechanisms, which are antibodies, cannot distinguish between "self" and "non-self," then the resistance of the body to invading organisms decreases, and infection and cancer may result. We see again the great importance of our understanding of the "self."

Carcinogens. Other agents known to result in cancer include a number of environmental and occupational carcinogens. A few examples include the following:

1. Chimney soot has been known to cause scrotal cancer.
2. Asbestos is known to cause lung cancer.
3. Uranium is known to cause lung cancer.
4. Cigarette smoke causes lung cancer, mouth cancer, bronchial cancer, and is associated also with bladder cancer.
5. Naphthalene dyes cause bladder cancer.
6. Vinyl chloride causes liver cancer.
7. Certain nitrates which are used as preservatives in various foods, especially meats, are implicated in stomach cancer and intestinal cancer.

Various drugs, including hormones, as well as immunosuppressive agents, some including those used in the treatment of cancer, will also themselves cause cancer. Radiation, such as that given off in a nuclear explosion or through exposure to x-rays, can cause cancer. So we see that a number of factors may be responsible for the development of this disease.

CURRENT APPROACHES TO THE TREATMENT OF CANCER

No completely satisfactory treatments exist.

Surgery: If the cancer, or tumor, is restricted to an organ or a portion of an organ, then sometimes cure can be effected by removal of the organ or removal of a portion of the organ. This happens only rarely. The procedure is often mutilating and can result in severe disability because of loss of function of the organ.

Radiation: Some cancer cells will die when exposed to radiation or x-rays in high doses. The problem, of course, is that radiation will also damage healthy cells and tissues and will cause sometimes devastating side effects and debility. In general, radiation will not cure cancer.

Chemotherapy, or Drugs: These are effective in a number of cancers. They are associated, however, with very severe debilitating and devastating side effects, such as loss of hair, sterility, impotence, nausea, and vomiting. Very often drugs will cure one type of cancer, only to cause the development of another kind. They make the patient more susceptible to the development of other cancers by causing immunosuppression, a term we have discussed previously.

Mind Technologies and Cancer

Medical research is discovering more and more about the mind-body connection in various diseases, and cancer is no exception. A rare but well-known phenomenon in cancer patients is that of spontaneous remission; that is, a person will recover from cancer for no known reason. Physicians dealing with cancer patients are very well aware of the fact that patients who have a strong positive attitude do much better than patients who have a negative attitude and a feeling of helplessness or hopelessness. In a study reported by cancer specialist Dr. Carl Simonton in *The Journal of Trans-Personal Psychology* in 1975, the attitudes and courses of 152 patients with cancer were studied. The responses to treatment were rated from excellent to poor. Twenty patients had excellent responses from the treatment. Fourteen of these patients were in very poor condition at the beginning and would have had less than a 50 percent chance of surviving five years according to all statistics. All twenty of these patients had what were described as positive attitudes. Twenty-two patients did extremely poorly. All of them had *negative* attitudes. Positive and negative attitudes are basically extensions of positive and negative thought processes. Positive attitudes and thoughts are those that generate emotions such as faith, courage, hopefulness, happiness, love, and belief. Negative attitudes or thoughts are those that generate emotions of fear, helplessness, hopelessness, and despair.

Various visualization and other mental techniques are being increasingly used as adjuncts in the treatment of cancer. Often patients are asked to visualize their disease, their treatment, and the body's immune mechanism. I saw a patient in my office who had come for a physical examination. She was an extremely bright, fresh-looking, youthful, vigorous-appearing young woman, who came for a physical prior to applying for a job. During the course of her history, I discovered that the patient had had non-Hodgkin's lymphoma, which is a cancer of the lymph glands. She had been advised to seek treatment at a prominent teaching hospital associated with a famous medical school in the Boston area. There she received the initial courses of chemotherapy. The cancer was extremely far advanced, being described as a Stage IV B, which meant that it included invasion of the bone marrow. The patient had extremely debilitating side effects from the chemotherapy and decided not to finish the full course of her treatment. Her father was a surgeon, her brother a physician, and she was under intense pressure from her family to continue chemotherapy treatment. Rather than endure the pressure, she left the country and lived in a small town in Europe for a year. There she practiced on her own, after reading a vast amount of literature on the Simonton technique, the visual techniques suggested by Dr. Simonton. A year later she returned to Boston. She had noticed herself the spontaneous regression of lymph nodes and abnormal masses in various parts of her body, including the armpits and abdomen. When she was seen in the cancer clinic of the same hospital where she had been previously examined, all the physicians were extremely puzzled at the complete absence of any evidence of cancer in this patient. They asked her what kind of treatment she had been undergoing and where she had been receiving chemotherapy. When she told them she had not received any additional standard medical treatment, but had been practicing the Simonton technique entirely on her own, the response of the doctors was typical of the establishment in general. They told her that this was a ''spontaneous remission'' and did not then further discuss why she had had a ''spontaneous remission'' or what exactly the term meant. Scientists and physicians quite often have closed minds and tend to dismiss an unexplained phenomenon with such terminology as "spontaneous remission." The fact was that this patient had been practicing a definite technique and, in her mind at least, there was a cause-effect relationship between the technique and the clinical response that ensued.

I recently had a patient with lung cancer who had an unusually good response to radiation and chemotherapy. This patient is still free from disease. She confided to me two years after she was "cured" that every morning she would sit down with her eyes closed and repeat to herself for about ten minutes, "I am going to get better, I am going to recover completely." She said that she actually believed that this would happen, and she had complete faith in these affirmations. She would repeat this procedure every day for at least fifteen minutes four or five times a day. She kept the fact of her practicing this technique a secret and did not tell anyone about it until several years later. This included me. Three years after her initial treatment she has no clinical evidence of the lung cancer.

Since then I have mentioned these examples to several of my patients, telling them that they should keep the fact that they are practicing such techniques to themselves and not speak to anyone about their practice. This is because I feared that negative comments from friends and relatives might diminish the effectiveness of the practice. I am convinced from my observations so far that these patients are doing much better than they would otherwise have done. I strongly recommend that they pursue radiation, chemotherapy, or surgery if it is considered necessary by an oncologist, but I believe that these mental techniques have a very important adjunctive role in their treatment.

I believe very strongly that there is a special kind of person who gets cancer. I am also convinced by my observations that cancer can be "licked," that it can be prevented as well as cured by establishing the right attitude of mind. We will explore the mysterious corridors of the mind and the mind-body connections in a later chapter.

The Role of Diet in Cancer, or the Diet-Cancer Connection

Although some members of the lay public have long felt that there was a link between diet and cancer, the medical establishment and scientific community at large has been very slow in studying and establishing the diet-cancer connection. Recently, however, a great many scientists have felt that there is a definite connection between diet and cancer. The National Research Council has recently issued a report entitled *Diet, Nutrition, and Cancer*. This report is 400 pages in length, apparently took two years to compile, and represents the most comprehensive review of the worldwide literature on diet and cancer published yet. The customary caution is that the evidence for the link between diet and cancer is as yet incomplete. The National Research Council has nevertheless issued the following dietary guidelines as a means of preventing cancer.

1. The proportion of calories from fats in the diet should be reduced from 40 to 45 percent, the typical intake of most Americans, to 30 percent. The Council has observed that the association between fat consumption and certain cancers, particularly cancer of the colon, breast, and prostate, represents the strongest cause-effect relationship in the entire diet and cancer field.

2. The Council recommends that people eat plenty of whole-grain cereals and lots of fresh fruits and vegetables, especially those high in vitamin C. The Council also recommends an increase in beta carotene, that is, an increase in consumption of dark green, leafy vegetables, carrots, squash, and vegetables in the cabbage family such as cabbage, broccoli, cauliflower, and Brussels sprouts.

3. The Council recommends that very little salt-cured, salt-pickled, and smoked foods be consumed. These include sausage, bacon, hot dogs, smoked fish, and ham. The Council has not yet recommended a vegetarian approach, but at a later point in this book, this new possibility will be carefully evaluated.

4. The Council recommends that alcohol be consumed only in moderation because of the high association of alcohol consumption and cancer of the mouth, esophagus, and stomach. Again, the Council is very cautious in making its recommendations, and still endorses alcohol

consumption in moderation. I believe that alcohol in any amount predisposes a person to a higher risk of cancer.

5. The report of the National Research Council also recommends against taking high-dose vitamin supplements, noting that toxicity from some of them, particularly vitamins E and A, can result. However, toxicity from vitamins E and A is rarely seen clinically and in my view supplemental vitamins have beneficial effects.

Vitamins A, C, and E probably play a preventive role in cancer. (The optimal doses for cancer prevention have not yet been defined). Vitamins C and E act as antioxidants and have been shown experimentally to detoxify certain carcinogens (chemicals that produce cancer). Vitamin A plays a role in inhibiting epithelial cell dysplasia. Epithelial cell dysplasia is a precancerous change in cells.

I commonly make the following additional recommendations to my patients regarding diet and cancer prevention:

1. Don't smoke.
2. Do not drink alcohol. Alcohol intake has been linked to cancer of the esophagus, mouth, and stomach.
3. Avoid excesses of hot coffee and tea, and "cola" drinks. Heavy consumption of hot tea has been linked to cancer of the stomach in Japan, and there appears to be a higher incidence of cancer of the pancreas among heavy coffee drinkers. (In some cases, heavy coffee intake has been defined as more than three cups per day.) Tea, coffee, chocolate, and the "cola" drinks are rich in methylxanthines. These are a group of chemicals that stimulate an enzyme called cyclic AMP in cells and make them more sensitive to the action of various hormones. Fibrocystic breast disease, a benign disease often confused with breast cancer, can be virtually eliminated by total abstinence from coffee, tea, "colas," and nicotine.
4. Avoid burned food, especially charcoal-grilled fish and meat. It has been quite conclusively demonstrated that there is production of carcinogens during charcoal grilling.
5. Include generous amounts of roughage or fiber in the diet. There is a correlation between colon cancer and the poor fiber content of Western diets.
6. Take optimal amounts of vitamins A, C, and E for the reasons mentioned above.

7. Don't eat too much—avoid obesity.
8. Avoid moldy and stale foods. Molds produce carcinogens.
9. Do not eat the same foods over and over again. Instead, use a variety of foods. Change your menu daily. Variety in diet is likely to prevent a high intake of any single carcinogen.
10. Eat a well-balanced diet and follow the principle of moderation in all things.

Additional recommendations regarding diet are made in the chapter entitled "Diet and Destiny."

From this discussion, we can see that a number of factors may be responsible for the development of cancer. However, these can be divided into the following major categories:

1. Outside agents, such as those mentioned above, including diet.

2. Intrinsic problems with the host, that is, the person who develops the cancer, which result in the increased susceptibility to cancer. It should be apparent that by and large almost *all* cancer should be theoretically preventable by, first, not being exposed to the inciting or causative agent, and second, by decreasing one's susceptibility, or conversely, increasing one's resistance to the causative agent.

Chapter Five

Cigarette Smoking, Alcohol Use, and Drug Abuse

If alcohol, cigarettes, and "recreational drugs" were eliminated from society, we would have nearly empty hospitals. A large percentage of people hospitalized for any illness can trace the source of their troubles to intake of alcohol, cigarettes, recreational drugs, or a combination of the above three.

SMOKING, SOME FACTS

1. Over 70 million Americans smoke.
2. Smoking undoubtedly is the major contributor to the two major killers, heart disease and cancer.
3. Coronary heart disease is fifty times more frequent in smokers than in non-smokers.
4. Lung cancer occurs eight times more often in persons who smoke one pack of cigarettes a day than in non-smokers; eighteen times as often in persons who smoke between one and two packs a day; and twenty-one times as often in persons who smoke more than two packs of cigarettes a day.
5. The death rate for cigarette smokers is 70 percent higher from coronary artery disease, 500 percent higher from

bronchitis and cancer, and 1000 percent higher from lung cancer.

6. Smoking is associated with a number of other illnesses, including duodenal ulcers, bladder cancer, cancer of the mouth and the esophagus, and also of the stomach.
7. So-called low-tar cigarettes often contain higher quantities of other harmful and toxic substances.
8. Smoking is a disease and warrants immediate remedial action.

ALCOHOL

No one any longer argues the fact that alcoholism is a disease. Alcoholics are subject to distinctly higher-than-average death rates. Persons with a history of heavy consumption of alcohol experience a mortality rate three times that of non-drinking people. The higher mortality rate results from diseases of the digestive system, suicide, automobile and other accidents, and homicides. Society and the medical profession have a different attitude, however, toward use of alcohol. In fact, some physicians have gone so far as to suggest that small amounts of alcohol may have beneficial effects. It is interesting to note that in a survey of people on the question, "What constitutes excessive alcohol consumption?" the definition of "excessive" was that which exceeded the respondent's intake. I believe that alcohol is a toxin, and that anything that impairs sensory perception or motor skills, even in small quantities, is harmful. I believe, therefore, that perfect health necessitates complete abstinence from alcohol.

RECREATIONAL DRUGS

Mind-altering drugs have been used since the dawn of civilization. Derivatives of *cannabis* (related to marijuana), hallucinogens such as certain types of mushrooms (*amanita muscaria*), soporifics, and stimulants have found their way into the tradition of almost every culture and every nation. The list of mind-altering drugs is too long to enumerate here—almost every substance in some way or other affects the mind.

The term "recreational drugs" is usually used to connote those substances which are frequently used to enhance, distort, or otherwise affect perception. The reason why a person initially resorts to the use of a recreational drug is that it gives him a "pleasurable sensation." The most frequently used drugs in our society today are alcohol, opiates (morphine, codeine, heroin), marijuana, cocaine, and occasionally drugs such as mescaline and LSD. A recent discovery which has fascinated scientists is that the human brain is capable of synthesizing chemicals very similar to opiates. These are called endorphins (end = endogenous, from within the body, orphins = morphine). These endorphins, or endogenous opiates, are the body's pain-relieving chemicals, and are, in fact, much more powerful than the exogenous compounds available at the drugstore.

Recent investigations have also uncovered the fact that the brain has distinct cells or receptors for the endorphins. Exogenous opiates must therefore exert their effects on the brain by binding to these same receptors. The very fact that these receptors have evolved bears testimony to the fact that there must be some use for the endorphins. However, since the brain and perception can be affected by a number of chemicals (such as, for example, alcohol, barbiturates, nicotine, amphetamine, mescaline, marijuana, cocaine, LSD, caffeine), it must mean that there exist in the brain receptors for these substances or for substances analogous to these chemicals (also called analogues). In other words, we must all be capable of synthesizing to some extent analogues of various types of mind-altering chemicals—otherwise, we would not have evolved the receptors to bind them. This idea may offer a clue to the perplexing problem of why people have since time immemorial sought after and experimented with mind-altering drugs.

Perhaps the organism is meant to experience altered states of consciousness. Nature has provided us with endogenous chemicals as well as receptors for these chemicals so that we can indeed experience and induce these altered states of consciousness. It may be that when our quota of these states is not ordinarily fulfilled, we tend to fill the gap with exogenous or pharmacological analogues.

The pharmacological analogues, however, not having been designed by the infinite wisdom of our body, have their toxicity. The recent increased use of these drugs has brought to light the fact that toxicity accompanies the use of almost every one of them. For example, marijuana, which until recently was felt to be relatively safe, has been shown to affect the immune system. Tetrahydrocannabinol, the principal active ingredient in marijuana, seems to localize in high concentrations in the spleen—an important site for the manufacture of T-lymphocytes. T-lymphocytes are believed to play an important role in protecting the body from cancer as well as infections. The T-lymphocytes in pot smokers are less able to fight back against an infection or a cancer cell. There are not only fewer T-lymphocytes present in these people; they are also very sluggish and slow to divide when facing an enemy force, e.g., infection.

In one study performed by Dr. Nahas at Columbia University's College of Physicians and Surgeons, the antibody production of pot smokers went way down during the month of heavy pot smoking; but what was surprising was the fact that production was just as off during the following five-week washout period when no pot was smoked. This meant that, in the case of heavy pot smokers, antibody production was definitely impaired and did not return to normal all that quickly. "After a potless five weeks, it was still significantly out of whack." Unfortunately, data such as this on the effects of marijuana on the immune system has not received the attention and publicity that it deserves.

Recently we have seen a national hysteria over a disease called AIDS (acquired immune deficiency syndrome). A disproportionately large number of people with AIDS were drug addicts. Although the evidence for the immunotoxicity of drug addiction is most striking in the case of marijuana, it is becoming obvious that immunosuppression accompanies the use of other drugs as well. Unless we quickly do something to change the trend in our society to continually experiment with "recreational drugs," we will be faced with the frightening potential of a major segment of our country's population being rendered highly susceptible to disease.

Because so-called recreational or mind-affecting drugs also impair sensory perception and motor skills, they are harmful. I do not feel it is necessary to belabor the point that drug abuse is responsible for devastating effects on our youth and society in general. It contributes to crime, accidents, suicide and homicide.

If we are to tackle the problems of cigarette smoking, alcohol and drug abuse, we must once again look to the mind of man. Why do some people crave these mind-altering stimuli? Could one substitute other mind-altering stimuli that are not harmful, but indeed useful and health-promoting? The answer is an unequivocal *yes*. There are mind technologies much more enjoyable and much more pleasurable that could be substituted for mind-altering drugs and alcohol, and that could result in positive effects on both mind and body. We will explore these technologies in the second and third sections of this book.

Chapter Six

The Problem of Weight Control and Obesity

Obesity is the most common metabolic disorder in affluent countries. A person may be said to be obese when his weight is more than 10 percent over his ideal body weight. One simple way of calculating ideal body weight is as follows: for men of medium frame, standard weight is 106 pounds for the first five feet of height and 6 pounds for each subsequent inch. One can add or subtract 10 percent for large and small frames, respectively. For women, a rough estimate is 100 pounds for the first five feet, and five pounds for each inch thereafter. Again, one can add or subtract 10 percent for large and small frames, respectively. Thus, a man of medium frame, 5 feet 8 inches tall, should weight about 106 plus 48, or 154 pounds. A woman the same height should weigh about 100 plus 40, or 140 pounds. If a person weighs more than 10 percent over his ideal weight, then he is obese or "fat."

Obesity is not only unattractive; it is unhealthy, and predisposes one to a number of illnesses. It has been definitely linked to the following problems:

1. *Heart.* Increased demand is placed on the heart when there is the additional need of supplying blood to excess body mass. Obesity is known to be associated with enlargement of the heart and certain diseases of the heart, including cardiomyopathy, a heart illness of unknown origin. Cardiomyopathy can lead to congestive heart failure, a condition where fluid backs up into the lungs, making

27

breathing difficult. In addition, there is an accumulation of fluid in the soft tissues of the body leading to swelling of the feet, and bloating and puffiness of the face. The left ventricular hypertrophy (enlargement of the heart) associated with obesity can be reversible if the patient loses weight.

2. *Joints*. Gouty arthritis is seen more frequently in heavy people. Gout can also be caused by certain "fad diets" where there is excessive intake of protein and limitation of carbohydrate intake. Osteoarthritis, or degenerative joint disease, is also more common in obese people. This can be particularly severe in the spine and other weight-bearing joints.

3. *Lungs*. Obese people display disturbed lung function as measured by sophisticated tests known as vital capacity and expiratory reserve volume tests. In addition, the oxygenation of the blood may diminish because of the disturbance in ventilation. Decreased ventilation (decreased air exchange) results from the effort required to move the chest wall. The decreased content of oxygen in the blood is responsible for the fatigue that is a common feature of obesity.

4. *Gall bladder*. Obese people develop gallstones with much greater frequency than people of normal weight. There is increased cholesterol secretion associated with obesity leading to increased formation of cholesterol gallstones. This seems to occur much more frequently in women.

5. *Diabetes*. About 80 percent of adult-onset diabetics are obese. Obesity causes enlargement of fat cells, or adipocytes. Enlarged adipocytes display resistance to the action of the hormone insulin, resulting in elevation of blood sugar, causing diabetes. Many obese diabetics who are currently taking medication or insulin injections could easily do without them if they lost their excess body fat.

28

6. *Arteries and Blood Pressure.* There is a higher incidence of atherosclerosis, or hardening of the arteries, among the obese. Angina pectoris, or chest pain from decreased blood supply to the heart, is more common in the obese population. There is also a greater risk of sudden death in these patients. The higher death rate of obese individuals may be directly or indirectly related to hypertension, which is more frequently present in obesity.

7. *Fatty Liver.* Obese patients have excessive accumulation of fat in their livers. If liver function tests are performed, abnormalities can be detected in up to 85 percent of obese patients. The "fatty liver" seen in obesity may be due to increased levels of a fatty substance known as triglyceride. Triglyceride is present in high concentration in the blood of obese patients.

8. *Varicose Veins.* Excessive weight produces increased pressure of blood in the veins of the legs. This causes distension of the vessels and subsequent incompetency of the valves in the veins. This incompetency can cause a condition known as "venous stasis" in the legs. Venous stasis in turn can result in thrombophlebitis (commonly known as phlebitis). Thrombophlebitis is a disorder where there is inflammation of the vessels, the veins, along with formation of clots in these vessels. Occasionally, these clots become dislodged and travel to the lungs, resulting in pulmonary embolism. If pulmonary embolism is massive, that is, if the clot is large, it can result in severe respiratory distress and sometimes even a fatal outcome.

9. *Surgical Risks.* Obese patients undergoing surgery have a much greater risk of developing problems from routine surgery. Anesthetic complications are more frequent in obese people. Surgery is also more technically difficult in obese people. There is also a higher incidence of postoperative atelectasis (collapse of the lungs), wound infections, and thrombophlebitis.

10. *Cancer*. Recently there has been a great deal of interest in the relationship of diet and obesity to the development of cancer. The diet-cancer connection is explored elsewhere in this book. There is evidence that obesity predisposes to cancer of the breast and uterus, especially in postmenopausal women. It appears that excess caloric intake stimulates production of the hormone estrogen, and it is the excess estrogen that is incriminated in the genesis of uterine and breast cancer. Obesity has also been shown to be a risk factor for prostate cancer in men.

How does obesity occur? Very simply, when caloric intake exceeds the energy requirement of the body for physical activity and for growth. I see patients in my office every day who come for help because they want to lose weight. They come to see me because they think they have a "glandular problem." Most of them do not. They simply eat too much. Most of them have tried various kinds of diets and lost weight in the past, only to regain it. They are frustrated and unhappy and come to see a physician, hoping he can find some glandular problem and cure them of their malady. Some of these patients do indeed have a hormonal or glandular problem such as an underactive thyroid gland or a pituitary tumor. If such a problem is uncovered, obviously the treatment becomes much easier. Therefore, it is important for a person who is unable to lose weight, despite going on a diet, to have a complete checkup, including some laboratory tests to rule out an endocrine, hormonal, or metabolic problem.

However, as I mentioned before, most people turn out not to have an underlying problem. If these people were to follow a diet, they would lose weight. There are any number of diets on the market, some sensible and some not so sensible. Basically their principle is the same—you must consume fewer calories than you expend in physical activity. I am not going into the details of these diets, since that is not the purpose of this book. All I would like to say at this point is that for a diet to be permanently successful, the person on it should enjoy being on that diet. In fact, he should not feel he is on a diet at all. He should eat a weight-controlling and healthful diet, not because he thinks it is good for him and will make him lose or control his weight, but because he would honestly not prefer to eat anything else. So once again, we begin to use words like preference and enjoyment. These are attitudes that reside in the mind, and I would like to emphasize that obesity originates in the mind and that its cure, therefore, will be in technologies that affect the mind.

Very often, one encounters the frustrated dieter's complaint, "All I have to do is look at food and I gain weight!" This may be literally true in many cases, according to many leading experts who deal with obesity. Research has shown that there are many people whose physiological make-up is such that they have a metabolic response to the sight, sound, or smell of food which is indistinguishable from that which is produced when food is actually consumed. In these people even the *thought* of food can, via the pituitary-adrenal-pancreatic pathway, cause a surge of insulin into their bloodstream. This rise in insulin can in turn cause irresistible hunger pains and speed up the conversion to stored fat of food that has previously been eaten. Insulin influences many of the body's organs to manufacture fat out of glucose and glucose by-products obtained from food. Experiments at Yale University have shown a dramatic rise in the insulin levels of overweight patients who were instructed to watch the cooking of a thick, juicy steak.

Dr. J. T. Cooper, author of *Dr. Cooper's Fabulous Fructose Diet* and past president of the American Society of Bariatric Physicians, urges dieters to make every effort to avoid the sight or smell of tempting food; they should cross the street rather than pass in front of a bake shop or candy store with a window full of goodies. When food commercials appear on TV, they should leave the room. He also advises dieters not to dine with normal-weighted people who appear to be able to enjoy all the fattening foods that are taboo items on the reducing regimen they are trying to follow. Every time they notice their minds wandering to thoughts of food, they should make a determined effort to think of something else.

Although Dr. Cooper's advice might appear extreme, it is in fact quite sensible. We see once again an example of the mind-body connection where our thought patterns literally dictate how we look, either thin or fat, and even how much we weigh.

Chapter Seven

The Problem of Chronic Fatigue, or That Tired Feeling

Fatigue, weariness, listlessness, languor, lack of energy, loss of ambition, absence of "pep," and weakness are among the most frequent symptoms found in patients in any doctor's office. These symptoms can occur in a wide variety of settings, including chronic infections, congestive heart failure, and debilitating illness, such as cancer. In these conditions, however, fatigue is not the primary complaint of the patient, but rather a secondary consequence of a more distressing symptom, such as, for example, shortness of breath.

Fatigue can be produced in any person by overwork. This can be physical overwork or psychological overwork. Chronic overwork without adequate rest will produce chronic fatigue. Persons with fatigue from too much work may not complain of fatigue as such, but may manifest the fatigue through other symptoms, such as restlessness, insomnia, and irritability. Chronic fatigue can have deleterious effects on an otherwise healthy person's physiology. Fatigue from overwork can lead to loss of a complex carbohydrate called glycogen from muscle tissue as well as to the accumulation of toxic chemicals such as lactic acid in the blood. It is interesting that the injection of blood from a fatigued animal into a rested animal will produce the manifestations of fatigue in the latter. This suggests that the symptoms of fatigue are mediated through the action of toxic chemicals released by muscles and other organs into the bloodstream.

There is certainly enough clinical evidence to indicate that the metabolism of patients with fatigue is altered by the fatigue. Such patients often have a faster breathing rate, faster pulse rate, dilated pupils, and higher blood pressure. Their blood count may show an increase in the number of white blood cells. All these physiological changes are the opposite of those seen in states of deep rest, such as sleep, and also in different states of consciousness such as meditation. People with fatigue also show decreased capacity for work, decreased productivity, inability to deal effectively with common problems of daily living, impaired judgment, poor ability to make decisions, and very often irrational, unreasonable, and irritable behavior.

When fatigue accompanies another chronic disorder, it is easily recognized as a secondary problem, and is not difficult to manage, since the management consists of treating the primary disorder. The problem arises when unexplained fatigue and lassitude are primary complaints and extensive investigation fails to uncover a primary illness. In these instances, fatigue is not usually an isolated complaint, and associated complaints almost always include nervousness, depression, insomnia, sexual inadequacy, poor appetite, headaches, irritability, and poor concentration. Patients admitted to hospitals with fatigue, or "exhaustion," are in the vast number of instances finally diagnosed to have either anxiety neurosis or depression. In one series, 75 percent of such persons were finally diagnosed to have anxiety neurosis, 10 percent to have primary depression, and the remainder to have a wide variety of psychiatric and medical disorders.

Several theories have been offered to explain the development of fatigue in otherwise normal people. Strong emotions, such as anxiety, can cause release of chemicals such as cortisol and adrenaline which may result in metabolic changes, which in turn lead to the accumulation of toxins in the blood. These toxins then cause the physical manifestations of fatigue. "Stage fright," a consequence of intense worry and anxiety, is an example of such a phenomenon. Strong emotion results in the sense of physical weakness, the inability to act, confusion, and finally exhaustion.

While this theory would readily account for the enervating effect of a strong emotion such as anxiety or worry, it would not explain the fatigue that frequently occurs in the absence of such strong emotions.

Some psychologists have suggested that fatigue is also a protective and self-preservative symptom which serves as a danger signal to the person experiencing it. It tells the person that something is wrong—that some attitude or some activity is too intense, too persistent, and must therefore be changed. Some psychologists have theorized that we all store in our minds a host of unacceptable ideas and notions. They further hypothesize that we repress these ideas with psychic energy, and that it is the depletion of the stores of this psychic energy that results in the physical manifestations of fatigue. There is another group of psychologists who feel that fatigue is not a self-protective mechanism, but simply the translation of an unconscious desire for inactivity.

Despite the above quite elegant and sometimes contradictory theories, some observations about fatigue are quite commonplace. Fatigue appears to be more common among people who seem to have no definite purpose in life. It is seen in people who have too much idle time on their hands, people who are bored, and people who are stuck in the monotony of routine. It is interesting to note that when these people are given the opportunity to "get out of the rut," and undertake a new enterprise or a new project, with a *definite goal in mind,* they snap out of their fatigue. Optimism and enthusiasm overtake them, and they forget that they were ever tired.

In my experience, boredom, lack of curiosity, and lack of enthusiasm are the most common causes of fatigue. These are attitudes that stem from the mind, and they are dealt with more extensively in later chapters.

Chapter Eight

Gastrointestinal Disorders

Disorders of the stomach and intestines are very common. Anyone who has experienced "butterflies" in the stomach or "knots" in the stomach during periods of stress or anxiety does not need to be convinced that the nervous system and gastrointestinal system are intimately connected. Indeed, the gastrointestinal system develops as an outgrowth of the nervous system during embryogenesis. In the adult, the entire intestinal tract is abundantly supplied by nerves through the autonomic nervous system. A number of hormones found in various parts of the gastrointestinal system, such as gastrin, secretin, cholecystokinin, gastric inhibitory polypeptide, glucagon, motilin, substance P, bombesin, and somatostatin have also been discovered in the nervous system. The exact role of these hormones in the nervous system has yet to be defined. It is sufficient to say that there appears to be a neuroendocrine-gastrointestinal connection that may have important ramifications, and that might further clarify the quite obvious psychosomatic nature of diseases such as peptic ulcer, irritable bowel, and various types of colitis. Emotional factors have been found to alter gastric function very profoundly. Many patients who have duodenal ulcers can often clearly point to an emotional upset that triggered the onset or worsening of their ulcer. Ulcers very frequently occur during periods of stress, and "stress ulcer" is a commonly-known disorder.

Irritable colon syndrome is the most common gastrointestinal disease in clinical practice. It causes a great amount of distress to patients and is most difficult to treat. The symptoms of this disease consist of lower abdominal pain and alternating constipation and diarrhea. Patients with this disorder are known to have markedly increased life stresses and manifestations of mild neurotic personality traits. Symptoms such as extreme abdominal pain, diarrheal stools accompanied by mucus, and generalized disability respond very poorly to any therapeutic intervention. However, when the severe psychoneurosis accompanying the abdominal complaints is treated, the gastrointestinal symptoms often resolve.

These are just some examples of a phenomenon we are increasingly seeing when we study any disease process in any system, and that is the phenomenon of the psyche affecting the soma, the mind (storehouse of thoughts), causing changes in body physiology, changes that ultimately result in the manifestation of a disease process.

Chapter Nine

Sexual Inadequacy

An increasing number of patients consult their physicians about sexual problems. Although in part this reflects a greater openness in discussing a subject previously considered taboo, it also in my view indicates a higher incidence of sexual dysfunction among our present generation. Sexual dysfunctions have generally been classified as either alterations in libido or alterations *in potentia*. In women seen in sexual dysfunction clinics, the most frequent complaints appear to be failure to achieve orgasm and lack of arousal during love-making. In men the most frequent complaints are premature ejaculation and impotence.

FEMALE SEXUAL DYSFUNCTION

Although no really good data exists on the various etiological factors responsible for orgasmic dysfunction, a number of factors do appear to play a role. These include, among other things, a negative parental attitude toward sex during childhood or traumatic experiences during childhood such as sexual molestation. An extremely common factor appears to be a negative attitude of the woman toward her partner, husband, or marriage. Frequently, the patient finds some aspect of her husband's behavior distasteful and is constantly angry at him. Often parental, societal, and religious injunctions deeply ingrained in the psyche of the patient produce inhibitions that interfere with sexual enjoyment.

Whatever the cause of the dysfunction, the end result in almost all cases is that the patient begins to focus on *evaluating her performance and the state of her arousal,* rather than just simply enjoying the act of sexual intercourse. The *evaluative thoughts* obviously interfere with the enjoyment of the act and inhibit orgasm. Orgasm is, after all, a *peak experience,* and peak experiences are possible only when thoughts are in suspension or have been transcended. In almost all studies, it is concluded that anxiety and over-concern about performance are ultimately the most common factors responsible for sexual dysfunction in women.

MALE SEXUAL DYSFUNCTION

Premature ejaculation, defined as ejaculation that occurs before either or both partners want it, is entirely a psychological problem. In their study of 186 men with the problem, Masters and Johnson concluded that premature ejaculation was "a learned reaction to early coital exposures characterized as time-pressured, guilt-ridden, or with fear of apprehension."

Impotence is the inability of a male to obtain or sustain a penile erection in the presence of sexual desire. It may occur in association with hormonal disorders, such as dysfunction of the pituitary, thyroid, or gonads. It is also frequently seen as a complication of diabetes. In the majority of patients, however, impotence is of psychological origin. Fears or phobias that arise about the sexual act, as well as feelings of guilt, are often responsible. Of all the psychological factors, however, a morbid preoccupation with ability to perform, or performance anxiety, seems to be the most common.

LOSS OF LIBIDO

In both sexes, loss of libido, defined as decreased desire for sex, occurs most frequently as a result of psychological or emotional causes. Frequently, however, decreased libido occurs as a result of the use of drugs such as alcohol, opiates, and marijuana. A common misconception among some people is that drugs increase libido and sexual potency. Drugs may increase sexual *activity* by removing social inhibitions, but the sexual activity is usually inadequate because of the depressive effects of the drugs on the central nervous system. To paraphrase Shakespeare, alcohol and drugs "increase the desire but take away the performance."

Depression appears to be the most common of all psychological factors responsible for decreased libido, but fear, insecurity, and guilt may also play an important role.

APPROACHES TO THE TREATMENT OF
SEXUAL DISORDERS

All successful approaches to the treatment of sexual dysfunction revolve around changing a patient's thinking patterns. A common technique is that known as "systematic desensitization." Since the dysfunction, in almost all cases, appears to be the result of learned habits of anxiety related to sexual participation, the technique attempts to eliminate learned factors in a step-wise fashion. The procedure usually involves three steps. First, the patient is taught voluntary muscle relaxation by any one of a number of methods (the Jacobsen technique is most popular). Next, the patient is asked to develop a list of hypothetical situations arranged on the basis of the degree of anxiety they elicit from him or her. The third and final step occurs when in a state of deep relaxation the patient is instructed to eliminate the anxiety. Visualizing each anxiety-producing situation apparently results, by a process of desensitization, in the ability of the patient to face the real life situation without anxiety.

The above approach has been used more frequently in the treatment of orgasmic dysfunction, but variations of the technique are used to treat other types of sexual dysfunction as well. Although these approaches are reasonably useful, treatment of sexual dysfunction remains largely unsatisfactory.

In my view, the increasing incidence of sexual dysfunction is a consequence of too much "cerebration" and concern about something that is natural, instinctive, and beautiful. Sex is one of the most powerful and spontaneous of all natural urges. Anything that interferes with the spontaneity of sex is bound to cause dysfunction. Until now, no human male has obtained an erection merely by willing it, and yet that is precisely what the majority of patients who seek treatment for impotence are trying to do.

The best way to approach sex is to leave it alone. When left alone and not dwelled upon, it begins to stir. My approach to the treatment of sexual dysfunction is frequently to forbid the patient or patients to entertain the thought or engage in the practice of the sexual act. While previously these same patients were totally preoccupied with, and yet unable to enjoy, sex, they now find the injunction of "leaving it alone" almost unbearable, and end up enjoying it spontaneously while trying very hard not even to entertain its possibility.

Sex is a wonderful and beautiful part of our lives. Like all other basic instincts, it has its origin in the mind. An innocent, open, non-demanding, loving, and giving attitude of mind can prevent sexual inadequacy of any kind.

Chapter Ten

Sleep and Insomnia

The sleep-wakefulness cycle that we are so familiar with occurs in all species studied by physiologists, although most scientific work has concerned itself mainly with the cycle in mammals. In mammals the sleep pattern is differentiated into two categories, Slow Wave (non-REM) sleep, and Rapid Eye Movement sleep (REM sleep). The phase known as REM sleep has been the focus of major attention among biologists, and it appears that this is the phase of sleep associated with dreaming. It is believed that this phase is responsible for the rejuvenation and rest that we derive from sleep. REM sleep has been described in birds, reptiles, and fishes, and is a characteristic that differentiates higher species from inframammalian vertebrates. In studying comparative and evolutionary aspects of sleep, one encounters the term "homology." Homology may be defined as "common ancestry." The common sleep-wakefulness pattern, as well as the morphological and functional characteristics of that portion of the nervous system implicated in sleep among all species, testifies once again to the fact that we humans are not isolated from the rest of nature, and that there is an interconnectedness, a homology and unity that binds us with all things in the universe.

The pattern of sleep in a human being varies during different periods of his life. Nocturnal predominance, or sleep mainly during the nighttime, appears as early as the first few weeks of life and continues

41

right through life. In extreme old age, this nocturnal predominance seems to suffer a progressive breakdown. A characteristic of the terminal years of life seems to be night awakenings of increased frequency and increased daytime napping in paroxysms or bursts.

It is not known how sleep produces its mysterious effect of rejuvenation. It is felt that fatigue produces a chemical substance (hypnotoxin), which activates a portion of the brain known as the reticular formation, which then mediates the sleep response. Of all the conditions that can result in a decreased sense of well-being and a compromise in efficiency, loss of sleep is foremost. If experimental animals are deprived of sleep for even a few days, they die. When human beings are deprived of sleep, they experience first fatigue, irritability, and inability to concentrate, and then disorientation. As sleep deprivation is prolonged, people begin to experience delusions and hallucinations, and there is a progressive decline in the ability to perform motor tasks. Further deprivation of sleep then leads to the appearance of signs and symptoms of neurological disease. These include weakness of muscles and problems with vision and speech.

Insomnia seems to be a very common disorder plaguing the Western civilizations, as attested to by the number of prescriptions physicians write for hypnotics and sedatives. (More prescriptions are written for this class of drugs than for any other.) Although insomnia can occur because of pain and various organic illnesses, the most common causes are nervousness, anxiety, and worry. In its most common variety, insomnia presents itself as a simple reaction to domestic and business worries. However, insomnia is also a frequent accompaniment of the more severe psychiatric disorders, such as major depression and manic depressive psychosis. In these more serious conditions, both the quantity and the quality of sleep are reduced. (By poor quality, we generally mean less of the REM sleep alluded to earlier.) A characteristic of depression is so-called early morning awakening, where the person has no difficulty falling asleep but wakes up around 2 A.M. or 3 A.M. and is then unable to go back to sleep.

Scientists and sleep physiologists have concentrated their research on the electrical and biochemical circuits involved in the induction of sleep. Much of this research has been utilized to develop sleep-producing drugs or hypnotics. These are of several varieties and range from simple relatively inert agents sold over the counter to more effective and habit-forming drugs, such as the barbiturates and recently a class of drugs known as the benzodiazepines. A characteristic of all drugs produced so far for the treatment of insomnia is drug tolerance; that is, they are no longer effective in the same dose after a short period of usage. Patients who take these regularly require larger and larger doses to produce the same effect. Another characteristic is that these drugs do not produce the right quality of sleep. Frequently, REM sleep is in fact decreased by these drugs. Alcohol, which can cause a stupor resembling sleep, also deprives the body of REM sleep. That the quality of sleep produced by these drugs is poor is attested to by the fact that people using the drugs complain of "hangover," fatigue, constipation, lack of energy and strength, decreased libido, and inability to recover from concurrent illness. Moreover, when these drugs are withdrawn, patients are in danger of developing delirium and hallucinations.

It is obvious, therefore, that current research toward the treatment of insomnia (aimed at developing newer and newer pharmaceutical agents) is misdirected.

It does not require more than common sense to observe that when one is unable to sleep, it is thoughts that keep one awake. Worry and anxiety are nothing but negative thoughts about something in the past and anticipation of some catastrophic event in the future (an event that probably won't happen). Sometimes, of course, we cannot sleep because of excitement about and anticipation of a happy event in the near future. We usually, however, do not mind that kind of insomnia because the sleep that is experienced after such excitement is usually very rejuvenating. Restful sleep is indicative of good health, and the quality of sleep serves as a useful index or barometer of one's mental (and consequently physical) health. Happy, contented, loving people never have insomnia. People ridden with anxiety, depression, and guilt never enjoy good and restful sleep. This has been known throughout the ages, and one does not need the support of science to verify this obvious fact. Sleep disorders occur in childhood only in association with severe painful illness or psychopathology. Children sleep well because of their innocence.

Any approach to the treatment of sleep disorders must begin with an understanding of thought processes. As with other illnesses discussed so far, it is to the mind, to the source of thought, that we must look for answers.

Chapter Eleven

Stress and the Burned-Out Syndrome

Stress is that which blocks the full expression of creative intelligence.

—Maharishi Mahesh Yogi

The word "stress" has been used very frequently in the last few years in connection with almost every disease from heart disease to cancer, to metabolic problems such as diabetes, and hormonal disorders, including diseases of the thyroid. It has become obvious in the last several years that stress is indeed a major cause of morbidity and even mortality. What exactly is stress? Several years ago, Hans Selye, M.D., introduced the concept of stress as the non-specific response of the body to any demand made upon it. He described what he called a "general adaptation syndrome" in which there was a predictable sequence of hormonal and physiological responses to any threatening stimulus. As the name implies, these responses evolved as protective mechanisms so that the organism could adapt to changing environmental conditions. Although Selye felt that all stressors, and these can be physical, emotional, or psychological stressors, produce the same sequence of physiological and hormonal changes, it is now becoming clear that this is not really the case.

Scientists now believe that the response of organisms to noxious stimuli is very individual and very specific. A standard definition of stress has emerged: "Stress is the accumulation of normal and abnormal pressures of daily living that test the individual's ability to cope." Dr. Daniel X. Friedman, an authority on stress, has defined stress in physiological terms: "Stress is a coupled action of the *body and mind* (my italics) involving *appraisal* of a threat, an instant modulation of response. The triggering mechanism is the individual's *perception* of threat, not an event. Perception is modified by temperament and experience. Response depends on the individual's target organ, previous level of arousal, and ability to adapt. Appropriate stress helps the individual to adapt. Inappropriate stress, however, serves no useful purpose and may result in disease." A very important part of this definition is that it is "the individual's *perception* of [a] threat," and not the threat itself, that is the triggering mechanism.

Let us take a few examples. Frequently-cited examples of stressors include divorce, loss of a loved one, loss of possessions, loss of a job, disease in a close relative, criticism by others. However, these really aren't the stressors. The stressors are the fear of divorce, the fear of the loss of a loved one, the fear of disease, the fear of criticism. Even imminent death itself is not by itself the threat, as is the fear of death. Thus, once again we come to ideas, to thoughts that excite biochemical and neural pathways, and modulate the stress response.

A large amount of scientific data now exists on the biochemical and hormonal changes that occur with stress. Cortisol, an adrenal hormone, rises in response to a wide variety of stressful stimuli. There are a large number of reports of the increase in cortisol during surgery. More detailed analysis of these reports, however, has revealed that it was the *anticipation* of surgery that caused the rise in cortisol rather than the surgery itself. Another hormone studied during stress was growth hormone. Elevation of growth hormone has been shown to occur among students during examinations, and during the viewing of violent or sexually arousing films, *anticipation* of *exhausting* exercise, and performance tests designed to provoke anxiety or distress. Other hormones that rise under similar circumstances include epinephrine, norepinephrine, and prolactin, a pituitary hormone. These examples illustrate quite clearly the psychophysiological connection—where a thought results in the secretion of a hormone which in turn causes a wide variety of metabolic and physiological changes in the body.

How does the stress response manifest itself? It manifests itself in the form of a disease process such as, for example, hypertension or duodenal ulcer disease. (There is a saying in medicine—"Ulcers are not what you eat, but what is eating you.") Or, stress may manifest itself with non-specific symptoms, commonly referred to as the "burned-out syndrome." The "burned-out syndrome" has received increasing recognition, and is characterized by exhaustion on all levels, physical, emotional, and attitudinal. Common physical symptoms are fatigue, insomnia, headache, backache, gastrointestinal problems, weight loss or weight gain, shortness of breath, or lingering colds. Emotional and attitudinal changes include boredom, restlessness, a feeling of stagnation, a tendency to rationalize, a tendency to feel indispensable, obsessive behavior, and depression. People suffering from burn-out are irritable, unable to enjoy or compliment colleagues' successes, generally cynical, defensive, fault-finding, and often dependent on alcohol and drugs.

One of the most striking recent discoveries about stress has been the finding of its deleterious effects on the immune system. It seems that in chronic stress, there is inhibition of the production of cells in the body known as T-lymphocytes and macrophages. This inhibition may be the result of excessive secretion of hormones, such as cortisol, as well as other chemicals seen in stressed individuals. T-lymphocytes and macrophages are natural killer cells and are responsible for protecting the body against infection as well as cancer. So one can see here a connection between stress and the development of diseases such as pneumonia and cancer.

Such are the myriad manifestations of the stress response. The key to all these manifestations, however, lies in the one place this book is all about, and that is the mind of man, where thoughts and ideas arise. It is to the mind and mind alone that all therapeutic strategies must be directed.

Chapter Twelve

Depression, Psychiatric Illness, and the Psycho-Endocrine Link

A wide variety of major psychiatric disorders are known to be associated with characteristic biochemical profiles.

Major Depression. This is a fairly common disorder characterized by unpleasant mood and loss of interest and pleasure. There are often other symptoms such as loss of appetite, sleep disturbance, loss of libido, feelings of guilt, loss of energy, and sometimes suicidal ideas. Patients with this disorder often have dry mouth, constipation, and disturbances in control of temperature and blood pressure. A number of biochemical disturbances can be seen in patients with major depression, and, in fact, it will soon become a common procedure to do blood tests in order to diagnose this kind of depression. Some of these biochemical changes include: a) increased secretion of the hormone cortisol; b) deficient secretion of growth hormone; and c) deficient secretion of thyroid-stimulating hormone, also called TSH. A pituitary hormone, prolactin, is often elevated.

Schizophrenia. This is a psychiatric disorder of young adults. Patients with schizophrenia display hallucinations, delusions, disturbances in thinking, and impaired social functioning. Schizophrenia has often been termed psychic ataxia. ("Ataxia" normally means a loss of control of a fine movement—holding a pencil—although gross movement—the hand can grip—is retained.) In these patients, there is often extreme excitement, agitation, restlessness, and irrational behavior. Abnormalities have been found in several pituitary hormones, including growth hormone, gonadotrophins, which are the sex hormones, and prolactin.

Anorexia Nervosa. This disorder is seen in young women and adolescents. The patient is morbidly afraid of gaining weight and imagines her body image to be fatter than it really is. The patient therefore rejects food, even though she continues to lose weight. Sometimes the disorder alternates with bulimia; that is, uncontrolled binge eating followed by remorse and shame. This disorder also is characterized by biochemical changes, including loss of secretion of luteinizing hormone and follicle-stimulating hormone. (These are sex hormones in the pituitary.) There is also seen elevation of growth hormone, elevation of cortisol, etc.

These are only a few of the many kinds of psychiatric illness associated with biochemical changes. Numerous other such disorders exist. Psychogenic amenorrhea is a condition where emotional distress causes loss of menstrual periods. Psychosocial dwarfism is a disorder where children manifest delayed puberty and markedly reduced stature (approximately 50 percent of age norms) and retarded bone age. These children usually belong to emotionally deprived families. Growth hormone levels are markedly decreased in the blood of these children. When they are removed to an emotionally supportive environment they begin to grow rapidly, tending to catch up with their age norms. Importantly, the blood levels of growth hormone rise concomitantly with the clinical improvement. Other children displaying the "maternal deprivation syndrome" may exhibit apathetic, withdrawn behavior. These children avoid personal contact, appear insensitive to pain, and often inflict self-injuries. Intermittently, they display disruptive behavior and temper tantrums. The biochemical changes in the blood of these children reverse when they are treated in emotionally supportive environments by loving, caring, and compassionate people.

In all of these cases, emotions such as love, compassion, fear, anxiety, depression and excitement express themselves as alterations in the biochemical milieu of the body. A major controversy exists in medicine as to which occurs first, the emotional or psychiatric disturbances, or the biochemical change. In my opinion, the argument is irrelevant. It does not matter which came first, the egg or the chicken.

It is sufficient to know that the chicken may come from the egg, or the egg from the chicken. What we are seeing here is that there is, in fact, no duality, no *real* psychophysiological connection. We create the connection in order to understand the physiology. The physiology is, however, ultimately just an expression of thought processes and excitations of intelligence in the field we call "mind." In these illnesses, as in others we have discussed, we find the origin in the mind of man.

Chapter Thirteen

The Psychophysiological Connection—
Some Dramatic Case Studies

The psychophysiological connection plays a crucial role in the genesis of all disease processes. It also plays an important role in the outcome of many disease processes. The following case histories reveal some dramatic examples:

Case #1: A forty-two-year-old business executive called me to say that he had been having mild intermittent chest pain for several months. The description of the pain was suggestive of angina pectoris. (Angina pectoris is due to decreased blood supply to the heart.) He said the pain usually came on when he was depressed, anxious, or trying to "make a deadline." The pain did not occur when he exercised. This history suggested that the pain was due to spasm of the coronary vessels (arteries that supply blood to the heart) as opposed to a fixed narrowing of the vessels, which occurs in atherosclerosis (hardening of the arteries). I advised the patient to come to the office for a checkup. He got extremely upset, saying he had no time, and there was "no way" he could get away from his projects for even a minute.

However, the episodes of pain increased in frequency, and he finally came to the office. In the waiting room, he became extremely aggravated because he had to wait fifteen minutes and began shouting at my receptionist, telling her that he was an extremely busy man and had no time to waste, and that I should not have made an appointment if I could not see him immediately. When I saw him in the examining room he was extremely angry, and began by telling me that doctors thought only their time was important and had no regard for patients' time. After examining him, I informed him that he was probably having unstable angina pectoris, and that he should be admitted to the hospital for additional diagnostic tests.

When he heard this, he lost control of himself and began to rant and rave that this was impossible. I saw then that he was frothing around the mouth and beginning to lose color over his face, and at that moment he clutched at his chest and fell to the floor. It was obvious that he had suffered a cardiac arrest, and we attempted resuscitative measures, but to no avail. Twenty minutes after this patient walked into my office, he was dead. An autopsy later revealed what we had suspected—the patient had a myocardial infarct (heart attack), but his coronary vessels were clean. There was no obstruction as is seen when a clot is present. The patient had suffered a heart attack because of "spasm of the coronary vessels." This spasm in turn had been induced by his hostility, anger, resentment, impatience, anxiety, and feeling of indispensability.

This patient was killed by his thoughts in a matter of two minutes. (I have dealt elsewhere with the mechanism by which this happens, but basically thoughts of anger and hostility, anxiety and resentment, induce complex physiological changes through the release of hormones via the pituitary-adrenal axis, which can cause changes in blood pressure and heart rate, and even induce spasm of coronary blood vessels.)

Case #2: I was asked to see a forty-six-year-old patient who had been admitted to the coronary care unit of a local teaching hospital in the Boston area. The patient was a visitor to this country from India and had been attending a business conference in Boston when he suffered a heart attack. While in the intensive care unit of the hospital, he developed a series of life-threatening cardiac arrhythmias. Cardiac arrhythmias are abnormal rhythms of the heart which diminish its ability to contract and therefore pump blood effectively. The most serious arrhythmia is ventricular fibrillation.

In ventricular fibrillation, the heartbeat is virtually ineffective, and unless the patient is immediately resuscitated, usually by the application of an electric shock to the chest, death rapidly ensues. Ventricular fibrillation usually occurs when there is electrical instability of the heart following a heart attack. It can be due to a number of causes including decreased oxygen supply, a deficiency of potassium, and other metabolic factors. This patient had suffered several episodes of ventricular fibrillation and had fortunately "been brought back each time" by the application of electric shock. It was not clear why he kept having the recurrent cardiac arrhythmia. It was clear, however, that if these episodes kept recurring, the patient would not leave the hospital alive.

When I saw the patient, I learned that he was extremely worried about how he would pay his bill. As a visitor from another country, he had no hospital insurance, and he had heard stories from other people that "in America if you were hospitalized without medical insurance, you would live in debt for the rest of your life." He told me he would rather die than live the rest of his life in debt. I assured him that the bill would be taken care of and that in fact, unknown to him, his company had taken out a special travel insurance policy for him and his entire delegation. After he was given this news his vital signs stabilized, and he had no further episodes of ventricular fibrillation. He was discharged in three weeks and left the country one week later completely free of symptoms. In this example, fearful thoughts would almost certainly have killed this patient had they not been allayed in time. (I never did find out what happened to his hospital bill.)

Case #3: A thirty-five-year-old lawyer came to the emergency room of the hospital complaining of non-specific chest pain. After careful examination, the emergency room doctor reassured him that everything was all right, and the pain was muscular in etiology. He developed chest pain again when he reached home and returned to the emergency room. On this second visit to the emergency room, I was asked to examine him. His physical examination and electrocardiogram (EKG) were normal, but I decided to admit him for observation because of his severe anxiety. Twenty-four hours later, I found that there were indeed some changes in his EKG which suggested that he had suffered some damage to his heart. These changes had not been initially apparent when the patient came to the emergency room. When I told him this, he became very upset and angry and immediately informed me that he was going to sue the hospital and the doctors who had initially seen him "for their incompetence." Despite repeated advice to calm down, he spent the next two hours calling various lawyer colleagues and making arrangements for "a lawsuit that would teach these bastards a lesson.'' His blood pressure rose despite attempts to bring it down with medication. An hour later, while still on the telephone, he had his third episode of chest pain and died instantly. Autopsy revealed myocardial rupture—literally a tear in the weakened or damaged portion of his heart. Again, it was this patient's lethal thoughts that resulted in his rapid deterioration and death.

Case #4: A sixty-four-year-old insurance salesman with a history of heavy smoking came to me for a routine physical examination. He had no symptoms and felt perfectly well. Because of the history of smoking, I ordered a chest x-ray. The x-ray revealed a large lesion in the lower lobe of the left lung. Further tests revealed that the lesion was consistent with bronchogenic carcinoma (lung cancer). A retrospective analysis of an x-ray done five years before showed a small coin lesion in the same area as the present findings, suggesting that the cancer had been growing slowly over the previous five years. In any case, the patient had been totally free of symptoms up to the present time. Upon learning of the diagnosis, however, the patient's condition deteriorated rapidly. Within three days he was coughing up blood, and in three weeks he had a severe uncontrollable cough and shortness of breath. In one month, he died from the lung cancer.

This case history illustrates something I have observed frequently, and that is rapid progression of and death from a cancer *after the diagnosis of cancer was made*. It is almost as if *the patient were dying from the diagnosis of cancer rather than from the cancer itself*. This is the placebo effect in reverse. The thought, *I have cancer,* leads to the thought, *Therefore, I am dying*. The thought is then translated via the psychophysiological connection into the sequence of pathological changes that cause the rapid demise of the patient.

Case #5: A sixty-two-year-old woman was admitted to the hospital because of jaundice. It was believed that the patient had gallstones, and she was therefore taken to the operating room for surgery. When her abdomen was opened, we discovered that she did not have gallstones, but a gall bladder cancer. The cancer involved the entire abdominal cavity and also the liver. She was considered inoperable, and therefore without any further maneuvers the abdomen was closed up. While the patient was still in the recovery room, we informed her daughter of the diagnosis. The daughter insisted that we not tell her mother. ''I know my mother," she insisted. "She will die immediately if you tell her she has cancer."

Reluctantly we told the patient that indeed she had had gallstones, and that these had been removed. We reasoned that the daughter would tell her the truth when she returned home. We also felt that the patient would not live beyond a couple of months.

I saw the patient eight months later in my office. Her jaundice had cleared up completely, and she looked radiant and healthy. There was no clinical evidence of cancer. The patient still visits me periodically for routine checkups and is free of disease. On her last visit, she told me, "Doctor, when you admitted me to the hosptal three years ago with jaundice, I was sure I had cancer. I was so relieved when you found those gallstones at surgery that *I made up my mind never to be sick again.*"

This is one of the most amazing cases I have ever encountered. In this case the placebo was not a drug, but the operation. In actuality, of course, it was not even the operation, but the patient's thoughts after surgery that made her live.

Case #6: As a fourth-year medical student in India, I was assigned to do a clinical workup on a patient with terminal cancer of the pancreas. The patient was a seventy-year-old Indian villager. Besides being very ill, he was confused and somewhat awed at being in a large modern facility with sophisticated machinery and teams of serious-looking physicians in long white coats. The doctors who took care of him were academic, professional types who would spend an hour at his bedside with interns and residents, discussing the pathogenesis of pancreatic carcinoma and its varied clinical presentations, and would then move on to the next case, sometimes without so much as asking him how he felt. The interns and residents took competent care of his metabolic problems, but were too busy to spend any time talking to him.

As a medical student assigned three workups a week at that particular time, I had plenty of time to talk to the patient, and in a couple of days we became very good friends. I learned he was a farmer from a nearby district, that he had three grown sons who now looked after the farmland, that he had previously been a very heavy drinker, and that because of his drinking problem his family had forsaken and deserted him. When he had become ill, one of his sons had brought him to this university-affiliated hospital and left him there with the words, "You will probably die!"

The patient had felt bewildered in the hospital, and now without the numbing effect of alcohol, he suddenly became aware of the searing pain in his abdomen and realized how sick he really was. His condition deteriorated rapidly, and his pain became worse. He found the doctors more interested in his disease than in him, and with no family to comfort him, he soon began to wish he would die.

I would spend an hour or so with him every evening, often without much exchange in the way of words. It was very clear to both of us that he had very little time left. My clinical rotation came to an end, and I was assigned to a "village posting" at a small dispensary about two hundred miles away. I went to wish him good-bye, knowing very well that he would not be alive when I returned to the hospital in a month.

However, I kept a stiff upper lip and said to him, "Mr. Govindass, I will see you when I come back in thirty days."

He smiled sadly and said, "Now that you are leaving, I have nothing to live for, and I will die." He was moribund and emaciated and weighed no more than seventy-five pounds. It was a wonder he was alive.

"Don't be silly!" I muttered, not knowing what else to say. "You cannot die before I see you again!"

I left for my village posting. The dispensary to which I had been assigned my rotation was understaffed, and I was busy doing the work of four people. I am ashamed to say that I seldom thought of my dying friend in the hospital, and when I returned four weeks later, I had almost completely forgotten about him. When I saw the name Laxman Govindass outside the ward, my heart started beating violently, and I broke out into a cold sweat. I could not believe that he was still alive. I rushed to his bedside. The old man lay crouched in bed in a fetal position. He was merely skin and bones, and the most striking aspect of him was the large bulging eyes that glared at me and looked deep into the innermost recesses of my soul.

"You have come back," he said. "You said I could not die without seeing you again. I am seeing you now!" He closed his eyes and exhaled his last breath.

I was deeply shaken. I could not forgive myself for having prolonged this man's agony and misery. I felt guilty and wretched, and
many a night I would wake up and find myself staring into his accusing
eyes.

I will never forget Laxman Govindass. It was through him that I
first stumbled upon the psychophysiological connection.

Case #7: I had just started my practice in a community twenty
miles north of Boston. I had joined a group of internists, two of whom
were sub-specialists in cardiology. It was a Sunday evening, and I was
on call covering for all my partners. I was driving from one hospital
where I had just finished my rounds to another about five miles away
when I received a call on my beeper to immediately call a Mrs. Johnson*
at a certain extension in one of the large teaching hospitals in Boston.
There was a sense of urgency in the voice of the operator, so I got to
the nearest public telephone and dialed the number. The voice at the
other end was hysterical.

"Dr. Chopra," she said, "my husband is booked for a coronary
bypass operation at this hospital tomorrow, and he wants to sign himself
out!" I learned that Mr. Johnson* was a patient of one of my senior
partners, a cardiologist. He had been having unstable angina pectoris
and had been transferred to the Boston hospital for emergency coronary
bypass graft procedure, since it was feared that he might suffer a massive
heart attack if the operation were not performed immediately. The hospital to which he had been transferred was one of the most famous in
the world, and the surgery was to be performed by a world-renowned
cardiac surgeon.

"Why does he want to sign himself out?" I asked Mrs. Johnson.

"Because he didn't like Dr. B. (the cardiac surgeon)." she responded.

"What did he not like about Dr. B.?" I inquired.

To which she replied, "Nothing in particular. He just didn't like
him."

*Not a real name.

"Mrs. Johnson," I said impatiently, "Dr. B. is a very competent and famous surgeon. People from all over the world come to Boston to have surgery performed by him. The hospital your husband is in is one of the best in the world. Sheiks from the Middle East, heads of state, movie stars from Hollywood, all come there for treatment. The mortality from surgery for the procedure your husband is going to have is less than one percent. Without surgery the prognosis is dismal, since your husband is having unstable angina and is bound to develop a severe heart attack, the mortality from which is very much higher. If your husband wants to sign himself out, that is his business, but he should have a better reason than the fact that he did not like Dr. B.!"

Mrs. Johnson replied, "Doctor, would it be possible to speak to Dr. A.?" (my senior partner, the cardiologist). "You see, he knows Mr. Johnson and he would listen to him. Mr. Johnson has nothing against Dr. B. In fact, Dr. B. was very nice to him and explained the surgery and everything very patiently. It is just that Mr. Johnson did not like his personality—nothing in particular, you know; it is just a feeling."

I was running out of dimes; besides, I had to get to the emergency room of the other hospital. I could not understand what she was trying to say.

"Mrs. Johnson," I said impatiently, "It is Dr. A.'s night off; I think he is away for the weekend anyway. I think your husband is pretty lucky to be at that hospital under such excellent care. Dr. A. went to a great deal of trouble to arrange for this surgery, and I think your husband should go through with it—or else he will almost certainly be in big trouble. If you will excuse me now, I have to hang up. I have to attend to an emergency."

The next morning I reported to my senior partner my conversation with Mrs. Johnson. As I was telling him the story, he began to run toward the telephone. "Where are you going?" I inquired.

"I am going to call off the surgery," he said. "Deepak, you will learn—never send a patient to surgery if he does not trust his surgeon." He remained on the phone for a while and then hung up. "Too late, too late," he said, "he's already in the OR (operating room)."

That evening my senior partner received a phone call from the surgeon. An unforeseen and very rare complication had occurred as they were getting ready to take Mr. Johnson off the cardiac pump, and despite very vigorous attempts at resuscitation Mr. Johnson had died on the operating table.

Case #8: Mr. K., a fifty-four-year-old businessman, was admitted to the hospital for the third time in three years with a bleeding duodenal ulcer. Careful review of his history revealed that all three episodes of bleeding had occurred during the month of April. Further questioning revealed that the patient had a "very stressful time in April every year because of income taxes." It turned out that Mr. K., like everybody else, did not enjoy paying taxes. It also turned out that he would make a "few justifiable adjustments" here and there that would cut his tax bill by a few thousand dollars, enough to save him some money, but also enough to cause feelings of guilt, unhappiness, and apprehension. In fact, Mr. K's unhappiness with himself was so strong he had begun to digest himself. When the obvious cause of his bleeding ulcer was explained to him, Mr. K. decided it was "not worth it." He turned over his tax affairs to his accountant and asked him to make contributions to the government on a regular basis throughout the year without resorting to any cheating of any kind. Since then Mr. K. has paid a few thousand dollars more in taxes, but he has saved several thousand dollars in hospital bills, and his health is greatly improved.

The relationship between duodenal ulcer and stressful life events has long been known, but only recently has the relationship between *anxious thoughts* and the secretion of acid in the stomach been recognized. In a very interesting article published in the journal *Gastroenterology* in January of 1983, Drs. Michael N. Peters and Charles T. Richardson evaluated two patients with symptomatic gastric ulcer disease who dated the onset of their illnesses to stressful events in their lives.

In the case of one patient, six family members had recently died, and the patient feared that he too would die soon. The other patient had been accused of grand theft, was under police surveillance, and had lost his job. Both patients had markedly increased gastric acid secretion rates, as measured by laboratory tests. These increased rates of acid secretion decreased to normal after hospitalization and reassurance in the first case, acquittal in the second case. Ulcer symptoms subsided at the same time as the decrease in acid secretion. This led the authors to conclude that the severe emotional stress in these patients led to acid hypersecretion and subsequently to ulcer disease.

In an accompanying editorial in the same journal, Dr. Herbert Weiner of the Neuropsychiatric Institute Center for Health Sciences, Los Angeles, California, asks,

> Why has the association of meaningful events and the onset of peptic ulcer resisted confirmation? The main reason is probably that we do not know the pathogenic mechanism that links experience with peptic ulceration, and therefore we disbelieve that such an association could exist. Another reason is that investigators seek a common series of events or a single emotional response that perturbs all such patients' lives. As this report indicates, however, the first patient had lost six relatives in short order, and also developed a fear of dying. The second patient was the subject of arrest, threatened with criminal prosecution, and lost his job. He was resentful, angry, and anxious. Only one common theme runs through these apparently disparate series of events—the loss of relatives or a job, *but it is not the event per se that is the central factor, but rather it is the meaning of the event to the person who experiences it. No test instrument has yet been devised that obtains reliable information on the meaning of an event to a person.*

Chapter Fourteen

All Sickness Originates in One Place

By now the reader should be aware of the hypothesis I am developing. The evidence is unmistakable. We have dealt with common problems such as high blood pressure, heart disease, cancer, weight problems, chronic fatigue, depression, burned-out syndrome, and psychiatric illness, and have found that the mind has an essential role to play in the genesis of all these disorders. This, in my opinion, is also true of any other disease that one cares to look at. Ulcers occur in uptight, anxious people. Irritable bowel, a common gastrointestinal disorder characterized by abdominal pain, nausea, and diarrhea, is considered a psychosomatic disorder. Ulcerative colitis occurs in people who are often very compulsive and obsessive. Impotence and other sexual problems are almost always due to performance anxiety. Accidents happen most often to accident-prone, absent-minded people.

These are only some examples of the psychosomatic relationship. As we probe deeper into the pathogenesis of disease, however, we discover that *all disease* results from the disruption of the expression of intelligence. This expression may be at the subcellular level, the cellular or tissue level, or at the level of the central nervous system. Enzymes, receptors, antibodies, hormones, and neurons are expressions of intelligence. While these expressions of intelligence are localizable, intelligence itself is not. It permeates each level of its expression, and is all-pervasive, universal, and cosmic. Intelligence is Mind, and Mind (as we shall see later) does not operate from within the confines of the brain alone. In that sense, all disease processes originate in the Mind.

So also does health.

61

Part II
Laying the Foundation

Let noble thoughts come to us from every side.
—Rig Veda

Chapter Fifteen

Happiness—Brain Chemistry of Health

The purpose of life is the expansion of happiness.
                    —Maharishi Mahesh Yogi

It is quite obvious that healthy people are happier than unhealthy people. What is now becoming increasingly evident is that the reverse is also true—happy people are healthier than unhappy people. It seems happiness (which simply means happy thoughts most of the time) results in biochemical changes in the brain, which in turn have profound beneficial effects on body physiology.

In contrast, sad or depressing thoughts produce changes in brain chemistry that have a detrimental effect on body physiology. Thoughts produce changes in the neurotransmitter content of the brain. At least thirty different neurotransmitters have been identified in brain tissue. The ratio of various neurotransmitters to each other can be changed according to the mood a person cultivates. Since thoughts are entirely under a person's control (you can consciously choose to think a particular thought), it becomes obvious that brain chemistry can be controlled very easily. This chemistry influences the content of various hormones from such areas as the hypothalamus and pituitary, and these hormones in turn have effects on distant organs in the body.

We could take a few obvious examples: erotic thoughts result in penile erection; angry, hostile thoughts can cause rapid heart rate, a rise in blood pressure, flushing of the face. Anxious thoughts can also cause changes in heart rate and blood pressure, in addition to tremor of the hands, a "knot" in the stomach, a "sick feeling," and sometimes an increase in the motility of the gastrointestinal tract resulting in diarrhea. Different kinds of thoughts must therefore produce different kinds of chemical changes in the brain. To quote a brain researcher, "There is no twisted thought without a twisted molecule."

Likewise, happy thoughts, loving thoughts, thoughts of peace and tranquility, thoughts of compassion, friendliness, kindness, generosity, affection, warmth, and intimacy all produce a corresponding state of physiology through the flux of neurotransmitters and hormones in the central nervous system. Scientists are now discovering that thought patterns can profoundly affect a person's health by releasing these chemical agents which have dramatic effects on body physiology. It seems that happy, pleasant thoughts produce good health because they are mediated by neurotransmitters that have a stimulating effect. Thoughts of enmity, animosity, hostility, anger, resentment, antipathy, strife, conflict, combativeness, gloom, and resentment may produce chemicals that reduce the body's immune capabilities and the ability of the body to resist disease.

The fact that thoughts can determine the outcome of a disease process is dramatically illustrated through the use of placebos. Curative results from placebos have been noted in a number of disease processes. A placebo is a pill or capsule that is made of nothing but sugar and some inert coloring to make it look like an authentic drug. In one recent study, one group of patients with bleeding ulcers was given a drug that was described as the latest, most effective medicine for the treatment of bleeding ulcers. Over 70 percent of the patients responded to the drug by immediately ceasing to bleed from the ulcers. Another group of patients was given the same drug and told that it was a new experimental medicine being tested. Only 25 percent of these patients were helped. The drug in question was no drug at all, but a placebo. Dr. Arthur K. Shapiro, a prominent researcher, states, "Placebos can have profound effects on organic illnesses including incurable malignancies." In the words of Norman Cousins, "The placebo, then, is not so much a pill as a process . . . The placebo is the doctor who resides within."

Placebos work through the release of neurotransmitters. In reality it is not the placebos that are working, of course, but the *thoughts* the patient has when he is ingesting the placebos. In the study mentioned above, the bleeding from ulcers was stopped by the thought, or belief, that the pill would stop the bleeding. Likewise, believing that a pill would cure headaches, relieve pain, lower blood pressure, improve sexual performance, increase strength and vitality, improve appetite, cause weight loss or weight gain, or even cure a malignancy, could have those corresponding effects. Thoughts indeed regulate brain chemistry, and the longer a particular pattern of thought is entertained, the greater is the effect of a particular neurotransmitter on brain physiology.

If thought patterns and the state of mind are so important, how can we change them for the better? To be able to do so, we must first understand what a thought is and what we mean by mind. This is the subject of the next chapter.

Chapter Sixteen

The Mind of Man—Reservoir of Intelligence
Thoughts—Impulses of Intelligence

The book you are reading at the present moment is nothing but an outpouring of thoughts from my mind streaming through your senses into your mind. Look around you, and you will see thoughts in manifestation. The chair you are sitting on had its origin as a thought, as did the house or apartment you live in, the bed you sleep in, the car you drive, the food you eat, the clothes you wear, the work you do. Let there be no argument about this obvious fact: all man-made objects, houses, highways, automobiles, jet planes, spaceships, computers, books, whatever you can perceive around you, are nothing but thoughts in manifestation, some your own, some other people's, but thoughts nevertheless. Maharishi Mahesh Yogi, a great Eastern scholar and founder of the TM Movement, calls thoughts "impulses of creative intelligence." These impulses originate in the mind or consciousness (the reservoir of intelligence), and if organized enough lead to creative action, and we have then the outward manifestation of the impulses of creative intelligence, an object of creation.

Let us take an example: I am an artist. Impulses of intelligence streaming out of my consciousness, my mind, when organized enough, lead to an action—the gathering of raw materials, such as paint brush and coloring materials, and then the mixing of them in an organized manner which results in an object of creation, a painting. In order for the painting to appear on the scene, a few things are necessary: a) consciousness or mind from which will arise . . . b) thoughts or impulses of creative intelligence in an . . . c) organized manner leading to . . . d) action resulting in . . . e) the object of creation. The ability to organize thoughts or the "organizing power," Maharishi calls knowledge. Any creative activity is nothing but the expression of organizing power (knowledge). This organizing power is an inherent property of mind. In fact, we could define mind as that structure that has organizing power. Another of Maharishi's favorite axioms is "Knowledge (organizing power) is structured in consciousness."

What about objects that are not man-made, objects of nature? These fall into two categories: living objects, such as plants and animals, and non-living objects, such as earth, wind, fire, water. Let us consider them in turn.

Take any living organisms from a simple, single-cell organism, such as amoeba, to the most complex protoplasmic machinery, a human being. What we see again is infinite organizing power, knowledge. Take the case of an acorn. An acorn is nothing but the collection of information packaged in an organized compact manner, which, when put into action, the right soil, moisture, etc., results in the manifestation of a huge tree. Or take a single-celled, fertilized human ovum. This is nothing but a set of instructions coded on a molecule of double-stranded DNA (deoxyribonucleic acid) in an *organized* manner, the expression of which leads to the formation of a human being—an Einstein, perhaps, who could change the whole course of history by his *thoughts*.

Take non-living objects. Take a piece of rock, break it into its constituent parts down to the last atom. What do we see? We see organization. We see a proton or protons, and we see electrons and other elementary particles in *organized* relationship to each other.

The point I am trying to make is this. Everything we comprehend in the universe with our senses, that is, all material objects, man-made, non-man-made, living, non-living, are nothing but expressions of organizing power, knowledge. Knowledge is structured in consciousness, and consciousness, or mind, therefore, is the source of all *items* in space and time—in the entire universe. To quote a Vedic text, "I am That, Thou are That, all This is That, and That alone is."

This is an astounding fact to grasp and come to terms with. What we are saying is that the only thing that is real and tangible in the universe is knowledge or organizing power. This knowledge or organizing power has its seat in consciousness, and all the rest of the material world is not really real or tangible, but just an expression of consciousness becoming manifest in one manner or another. To quote Napoleon Hill, who has utilized this knowledge and provided a technology of success which is based entirely on the above concepts: "We look not to the things that are seen, but to the things that are unseen, for the things that are seen are transient, but the things that are unseen are eternal."

Let us restate what we have said so far, and express what we have said in more graphic terms. First, we have consciouness or universal mind, in which reside impulses of intelligence. These are expressed as thoughts in our mind, which, when expressed in an organized manner (organizing power or knowledge) result in all material creation. Our thoughts are the same as all the other impulses of intelligence in nature. We just call them thoughts because that is how we think of them. A bird taking a trans-Atlantic migrational flight also has an impulse of intelligence, leading it to the action which is the trans-Atlantic flight. That impulse in the bird's brain is in a sense also a thought, only we do not call it a thought because we are accustomed to thinking of thoughts only in human terms. Likewise, the impulses of intelligence that lead a worker bee to collect pollen from flowers and manufacture honey are in a sense also thoughts.

All of nature is therefore nothing but a teeming universe of all kinds of impulses or thoughts, expressing themselves in the infinite variety of creation.

So also when we look to our bodies, we see the same infinite intelligence in operation. We are used to thinking of intelligence as residing only in the brain. That is because we equate intelligence with intellectual ability and intellectual tasks, and because that is our frame of reference. However, with our new insight, we discover intelligence operating in every cell in our body. The intricate machinery of the heart, of the kidney, the immune or endocrine systems, all these are other expressions of intelligence or organizing power. We come to the inescapable conclusion that mind or consciousness, or intelligence, pervades every fiber of the structure of the universe. Our own minds are but one expression of this infinite intelligence.

Chapter Seventeen

Health, the Algebraic Sum of Positive and Negative Impulses of Intelligence

At any one moment of time, your health is the sum total of all the impulses, positive or negative, that emanate from your consciousness. Put another way, you *are* as you think. If you are happy, it just means your thoughts are happy most of the time. If you are depressed, it only means you have sad thoughts most of the time. So also with other states of mind, such as anger, fear, frustration, anxiety, greed, envy, love, compassion, hate, hostility, kindness, and benevolence. These are all simply thoughts. But when one of them is predominant, it leads to a corresponding state of mind and ultimately of body. If you are having hostile, angry thoughts, that is reflected in your facial expression, in your behavior toward people, and in the way you feel physically. Typically your face has a scowl, you are impatient and difficult to deal with, you churn up a lot of acid in your stomach and a lot of adrenaline from your glands, and you suffer from peptic ulcer and hypertension. On the other hand, if you have thoughts of love, peace, and compassion, these too are reflected in your demeanor, in your behavior, and in your health.

For an observant person, it is really not at all difficult literally to read your thoughts. These are written all over your face, in your actions, in your behavior, and in the state of your health.

In the enlightened person, and we will talk about the neurophysiology of enlightenment in a later chapter, thoughts are not the mechanical outcome of simple interaction between subject and object. Rather, the highly evolved mind has complete and total mastery over the thinking process. The potential for this exists in all of us, and with proper knowledge and organizing power we too can be totally in charge of how we feel, mentally and physically. Not only that, we can control our universe in any way we want, and thus unlock the secrets of a prolonged and ever-youthful life.

Chapter Eighteen

Evolution

A few years ago, an infinite amount of information packaged in a minuscule microscopic, flagellating, single-celled sperm was combined with an infinite amount of information packaged in a single-celled, microscopic ovum. The result was again an infinite amount of information now packaged in an infinitesimally small, single-celled conceptus. That single-celled conceptus with infinite information was unique because there was nothing else in the entire universe with exactly that set of instructions coded on its double-stranded DNA (deoxyribonucleic acid). With proper nourishment and food, that cell divided again and again billions of times, carrying with it all the time its unique knowledge and its unique packets of information. Today that cell is billions of cells working in concert with each other in a display of ever-intricate and ever-organized knowledge and intelligence. Today that cell is you.

It is all your thoughts, all your emotions, likes, dislikes, passions, and desires. Today you may be reaching for the stars, conquering the outer reaches of space, expounding a radical philosophy, or stirring up a revolution. You may be a Hitler or a Gandhi, and the face of the world may be changed forever because of you. Who are you? In truth, you are none other than that single cell, conceived accidentally, when one of several hundred million sperms carrying its unique set of instructions, surging ahead of its companions, entered an ovum in your mother's womb. The information you possess, that code of instructions on that double-stranded DNA, is the same today as it was then. You are just that set of instructions and nothing else. That set of instructions is *all of you*—your hair follicles, your skin, your genitalia, your eyes, your senses, your mind, and your intellect. You are *a piece of knowledge*. That knowledge continues to be expressed in infinite variety so that you are not the same person today as you were yesterday, and you will be another different person tomorrow. This is what we call evolution.

But evolution does not mean that you have really become different or acquired more knowledge. The knowledge was complete and whole to begin with. It was infinite, and it was contained in the single cell that you started out as. Only the expression of that knowledge is ever-expanding. Is there a limit to this expansion, to this evolution? No. Like the universe, the expression of this knowledge is infinite and unbounded. That is your potential—*infinite*. That is the claim that led Napoleon Hill to observe "Whatever the human mind can conceive, the human mind can accomplish." This is a very profound statement, and the realization of its truth is the key to all success. That is why it has also been said that "Nothing is impossible."

Chapter Nineteen

The Problem of Aging—Living, Longevity, Mortality, and Immortality

Aging may be defined as a progressive deterioration in physical and mental function that occurs with time, ending with the cessation of all function, which is death. The mechanisms of aging are not clear. Until recently scientists had not shown much interest in the aging process, and not too much research exists on the subject. However, the function of various organs has been studied, and there is only one way to describe aging—it is a progressive decline with time. Hormones also have been studied, and it has been found that interesting changes occur in the blood concentration of particularly the pituitary and adrenal hormones. For example, there is a rise in the blood concentration of a pituitary hormone called thyroid-stimulating hormone and a decline in the concentration of an adrenal hormone called dehydroepiandrosterone sulfate as people grow older. (I was involved in some of this research as an endocrine fellow.)

It is interesting to note that the technique of Transcendental Meditation causes the opposite changes. Long-term meditators show lower concentrations of thyroid-stimulating hormone and higher levels of dehydroepiandrosterone sulfate than control subjects, indicating that the experiences during meditation are somehow translated into biochemical messages that may reverse the aging process. (I will discuss the effects of the TM technique on the aging process in another chapter.) Along with the alteration and concentration of hormones is a subtler but more significant change in the expression of the hormones. This means that the same concentration of a hormone in the blood no longer has the same effect as it previously had, an indication that underlying the organic or physical decline is a nonphysical or functional decline.

In the last few years there has been some research on animals that may give us some clues as to the mechanics of the aging process. Whether the work done with animals is relevant to humans is hotly debated among scientists. However, since there appears to be a homology of structure and function among all living species, I think the experimental data offers some interesting insights into what may influence aging. Fasting has been a tradition in many cultures and a ritual in many religions throughout the centuries. It appears that this practice may in fact have some beneficial physiological effects. Experimentally, it has been shown that the life span of rats can be extended by periodic fasting. During fasting there is a rise in the level of pituitary growth hormone. One of the effects of growth hormone is the stimulation of the production of T-lymphocytes in the thymus. T-lymphocytes play an important role in providing immunity to an organism. Aging and age-related chronic diseases such as arthritis and some malignancies occur when the body's immune response is diminished. Physical exercise also raises the level of growth hormone in the blood. Objective science is thus supporting the claims of some lay people who have long maintained that regular exercise and regular fasting are life-prolonging measures. Levels of growth hormone also rise during sleep, lending support to the long-held idea that an adequate amount of sleep is necessary for a long and healthy life. Other factors that may raise the level of growth hormone in the blood are the amino acids arginine and ornithine. These are being touted as ''youth pills'' and are being sold in health food stores across the country. Age researchers Durk Pearson and Sandy Shaw, authors of the recent best seller *Life Extension,* recommend taking 500 mg to a gram of arginine or ornithine just prior to bedtime.

It is too early to tell whether these attempts at increasing levels of growth hormone through exercise, fasting, or dietary manipulation will really prolong a person's life span, although the initial data does appear very promising. It must be cautioned that periodic fasting should not be engaged in to the point of malnutrition. Protein-calorie malnourishment also leads to decreased immunity. By and large, dietary measures agreed to by most researchers in this field include a gradual reduction in the amount eaten, avoidance of processed foods, avoidance of foods high in salt, fat, and sugar, and an increased intake of fresh fruits and vegetables.

Another aspect of the research on the effect of diet on life extension has focused on antioxidants. It is felt that aging and age-related pathological processes such as atherosclerosis may occur due to the formation of free radicals in the body. Free radicals are formed in the body as a result of chemical interaction between the body's cells and environmental agents that are ingested in food or water or inhaled as polluted air or tobacco smoke. Oxygen is used up during these reactions. Antioxidants are chemicals that prevent the formation of free radicals. Many of these antioxidants are found in natural foods. However, many aging experts are recommending supplemental intake of antioxidants to combat aging. The ones generally available in health food stores are the vitamins A, C, E and pantothenic acid, the trace minerals selenium and zinc, and the amino acid cysteine. Frequently recommended doses are 2 grams of vitamin C, 600 international units of vitamin E, 25,000 international units of vitamin A, 20 milligrams of zinc, 100 micrograms of selenium, and 500 milligrams of cysteine daily. It must be cautioned that these recommendations are based on preliminary data and do not have the sanction of the medical establishment or the Food and Drug Administration.

Emotional stress and worry can hasten the aging process. Stress and worry mediate their effects through the neuroendocrine axis. Thoughts are translated into changes in the flux of neurotransmitters in the brain which in turn affect the concentrations of hormones such as ACTH in the pituitary. Excessive secretion of ACTH causes increased cortisol secretion by the adrenal glands. Increased levels of cortisol can adversely affect the formation of T-lymphocytes and antibodies and lead to immunosuppression and its associated diseases and pathological processes.

The fact that the central nervous system has such an important role to play in the aging process has led scientists to hypothesize that there is a biological clock in the brain which determines the life span of a particular species. According to this theory, the maximum life span is genetically determined by this clock in the brain, and environmental factors further modify this predetermined timing in the central nervous system. This theory leads to some very exciting possibilities. Since this setting of the biological clock is determined genetically, it should be possible through genetic manipulation and engineering to alter the expression of the informational content of the genes and re-program and reset the biological clock. Such ideas are stimulating the imagination of present-day biologists and genetic microengineers, who are now beginning to entertain the notion of immortality. In fact, techniques already exist to "immortalize" or make cells live forever in vitro (in the test tube).

Although this idea of immortality may seem novel to us, it is not new to nature. The lowly amoeba, a unicellular organism, is literally physically immortal. When it reaches senescence, its single cell divides into two younger, more lively and vibrant amoebae. The amoeba does not die; it becomes its two daughters. The younger amoebae, as they mature, do likewise. In this continued and everlasting propagation of amoebae the "original" amoeba remains, and no corpse is ever found. Another organism, the hydra, a cylindrical-shaped creature, has also discovered the fountain of youth and everlasting life. The metabolism of the hydra is so rapid that all of its body cells are replaced every two weeks. Its life expectancy thus remains a constant. There is no aging, and there is no death.

Nature's intelligence has programmed other cold-blooded species, certain types of fish and crocodiles, with such low metabolic rates that their cells are forever growing. These fish and crocodiles keep maturing forever and ever. There is no fixed adult size, and death as an event occurs only when they fall prey to other predators. Other life forms such as the redwood tree and the bristlecone pine may not be immortal, but are alive and well today at ages 4,000 to 5,000 years old. The Bodhi tree under which the Buddha meditated more than 3,000 years ago is a shrine and a place of pilgrimage in India today.

When scientists attempt through genetic microengineering techniques to "immortalize" cells, they are not altering the informational content of the genes, but merely the expression of the genes. Genes themselves have always known the secret of immortality. They are the one living entity within us that never dies. Mutations occur, of course, and the expressions of the genes may change through the millenia, but the genes themselves live on forever. This fact was brought home to me rather dramatically when my wife was pregnant with our first child fourteen years ago. A routine blood test had revealed that she was mildly anemic. I assumed she must have a mild iron deficiency, but out of curiosity I looked through a microscope at the slide prepared from a drop of her blood. When I saw the bizarre shapes and forms of the red cells I took the slide to the pathologist at our hospital, who promptly made a diagnosis of "mild Mediterranean anemia." A more sophisticated blood test (hemoglobin electrophoresis) confirmed that Rita had the thalassemia minor trait. Since thalassemia is a blood disorder common to Mediterranean people and my wife was born in New Delhi, India with no known relatives outside that area, I was even more intrigued. I took to the libraries and made inquiries of epidemiologists and researchers in India, and discovered that "a belt of thalassemia" existed all the way from Macedonia, Greece to an area called Multan in Pakistan. I learned that Rita's great-grandfather had migrated to India from Multan. I also discovered that this "belt of thalassemia" was more or less the exact route taken by the armies of Alexander the Great, King of Macedonia, centuries before the birth of Christ. As I sat there looking for the hundredth time at this little smear of blood under a microscope in a dingy laboratory in a small community hospital in Plainfield, New Jersey, in A.D. 1970, the reality of immortality dawned on me with a suddenness that exhilarated me. Those little genes, coursing through my wife's veins with gay abandon, had outlived all: Pompeii, the glory of Rome, Christ's Sermon on the Mount, the Crusades of the Middle Ages, the conquests and defeats of Napoleon, revolutions in China, France and Russia, the emergence of Darwin's theory of evolution, the colonization of the British Empire, the discovery of America—all these events had come and gone and those genes I was staring at had lived through them all. Through all the turmoils and upheavals of the centuries they had survived, and they continue to survive in my wife, and now my children. Surely, we need no more convincing proof of immortality; genes are living embodiments of everlasting existence.

Are genes physical structures, or are they simply unique expressions of timeless knowledge—impulses of intelligence? They are both. They are physical because you can see them and analyze their components in terms of chemical structure, but like other living tissue they transcend their mere physical structure. They are always and ever in dynamical relationship with the rest of the universe. They are ever the same, and yet every moment they are new. Genes are precipitated information. They are the physical expression in very concentrated form of "Knowledge" that has always existed—knowledge that transcends both space and time. If we are ever going to grasp this notion of immortality we must learn to experience this knowledge, not intellectually, but through direct cognition without the use of our senses. For our senses are tied up with this thing we call time, and time, in Krishnamurti's words, is "the psychological enemy of man."

Since aging occurs with the passing of time, we must have a clearer conception of time. What is it? Krishnamurti says "thought is time." Einstein proved that time is relative. We are now coming to realize that indeed time is a concept. Nobody has ever seen time, nobody has ever touched it, heard it, smelled or tasted it. It exists totally outside of our senses and only in our consciousness. We have created time, you and I. Time is an imaginary mental device, a concept we use to measure the relative motion of bodies in relation to one another in space. We also know now that we must no longer think of time as an entity unto itself, but rather as a partner in the larger space-time continuum. This better understanding of time is the key to our understanding of the aging process, since aging occurs with what we call "the passage of time." It was Einstein who first presented the notion that if you travel close to the speed of light, that is, 186,282 miles per second, you could slow down or "dilate" time. The English physicist L. R. Shepherd has calculated that if you could travel at close to the speed of light to a nearby star, a few light-years away, and come back in three years, that is, three years for you, you would find that twenty-one years had elapsed on the earth. In other words, although you might have grown only three years older, your friends and relatives on earth would have aged by twenty-one years. So we see that aging, too, could be a relative phenomenon.

Dr. Larry Dossey, a prominent physician (whose book, *Space, Time and Medicine,* I highly recommend) observes,

> . . . we cling to the idea of a real time—a time that flows and is divisible into past, present, and future. Our belief in a linear

real time underlies our basic assumptions of health and disease, of living and dying. But this kind of thinking is tied to an older science, which depended on an external reality, a reality independent of our senses. This view of the world has been discarded by modern physics. If we revise our idea of time in order to be consistent with the modern physical views, we must say of it what we have been forced to say of the external world: *time is bound to our senses*—it is part of us, it is not "out there." And our concepts of health and disease consequently must be revised, dependent as they are on our view of time.

Mortality, birth, death, longevity, illness, and health—we unconsciously construct these ideas, incorporating into them an *absolute* time, which we assume to be part of an *external* reality. But if Einstein was correct that all knowledge about reality begins and ends in experience, there is no external reality from which these events draw meaning. Our knowledge of health begins and ends with experience—i.e., health issues are quintessentially experiential; there is simply no other place to go for meanings of health, illness, life, and death than to our own senses. These events, thus, are not absolute.

What is being said here is that since the picture of the world out there is not really the look of it, but only our way of looking at it—*if we could only change our way of looking at it, we could, in fact, change all notions and all realities about living, aging, mortality, and immortality, for it is our notions that construct that reality, it is our ideas, our thoughts, that construct that material universe.*

Think of it for a moment. What is your body composed of? The tissues and cells that construct your physical body, including the immortal genes, are nothing but atoms and subatomic particles arranged in a particular configuration. The atoms and subatomic particles themselves are identical to similar atoms and subatomic particles that exist in the rest of the universe. They are neither created with your birth nor destroyed with your death. They have always existed as atoms and subatomic particles. They are part and parcel of the space-time continuum. It is only their arrangement that has resulted in the entity that is you. In fact, the body that is "you" is not even composed of the same particles or atoms today that it was composed of a few years ago, for the atoms composing your tissues, your cells, slough off and replace each other daily. In fact, you should not think of your body as a "frozen sculpture" with the same atoms and subatomic particles, but rather as a river. In the words of Heraclitus, "You cannot step twice into the same river, for new water is always flowing in."

The analogy with the river is particularly beautiful and very apt. In the novel *Siddhartha,* Herman Hesse expresses his fascination with the river when he says, "Love this river, stay by it, learn from it." Siddhartha "wanted to learn from it, he wanted to listen to it. It seemed to him that whoever understood this river and its secrets would understand much more, many secrets, all secrets. . . . today he saw only one of the river's secrets, one that gripped his soul. He saw that the water continually flowed and flowed and yet it was always there; it was always the same and yet every moment it was new. Who could understand, conceive this? He did not understand it; he was only aware of a dim suspicion, a faint memory, divine voices."

Your body is like that river—it is always the same and yet every moment it is new. Those atoms and subatomic particles that you think are you are the same subatomic particles that structure the rest of the universe. You are not absolute static matter. The carbon of your bones and the hydrogen of your plasma is constantly and ever in dynamic and actual physical exchange with all other bodies through the processes of respiration, digestion and elimination. The particles structuring the eyes that see for you today and the brain cells that record and store information for you today are in constant flux. They are the interstellar dust of yesterday and the trash of tomorrow. This objective truth of modern science is also the subjective cognition of the mystic who sees in this constant and everchanging flux of particles the cosmic biodance of Shiva.

So if your material body is not the real you, what is? The real you is the *arrangement,* the *organizing power,* the *knowledge,* the *intelligence,* the *impulse of consciousness,* that arranges those atoms and particles to give the appearance of you. That intelligence, that organizing power, that impulse, that thought, is the only reality. It is non-material, whole, non-changing, never born, never dying, immortal. Its infinite expressions result in the appearance of growth, evolution, decline, decay, death. That is your true nature. This realization of modern science has been intuitively grasped through the ages by many spiritually inclined persons and mystics. To quote some passages from the ancient *Bhagavad Gita*, "He is never born, nor does he ever die, nor having once been, does he cease to be. Unborn, eternal, everlasting, ancient; he is not slain when the body is slain. Weapons cannot cleave him, nor fire burn him, water cannot wet him, nor wind dry him away. He is eternal, all pervading, stable, immoveable, ever the same. He is declared to be unmanifest, unthinkable, unchangeable."

This unmanifest intelligence is the real you; you are in reality this non-material, formative force. Many scientists use the analogy of a field to describe this force: "just as a magnetic field can orient a pile of iron filings into a certain pattern, so this force can shape body and mind." Maharishi Mahesh Yogi calls it "the field of all possibilities." From this field spring all the impulses that are responsible for creation, evolution, and dissolution.

It is my belief that as we gain more and more insight into our true identities and our true selves, we will also begin to realize that the aging process may be an expression of ancient myths and ideas, and social prejudices that propel people into decline. These ideas, so entrenched through centuries of cultural conditioning and indoctrination, make up our belief system, and this belief system spawns the notion that the passage of time results in decay and death, a self-fulfilling prophecy. I believe this prophecy is mediated via the central nervous system, the ideas, the notions and thoughts affecting specific autonomic and sensory processes, which in turn relay messages to the body. I also believe that there is a way to change this, but first we must radically change our traditional viewpoints, viewpoints that are merely relics and residues of immemorial myths. Since the human mind can achieve anything it can conceive, it can by altering its viewpoints and its traditional notions and ideas change even the aging process, and make the idea of immortality a reality.

Chapter Twenty

Man and Superman

Man has evolved over a few eons of time from a single-celled organism to a creature of infinite potential. Today he stands on the threshold of even newer and bolder discoveries. The development of technology is one of the most impressive and striking pieces of evidence of man's creative capabilities. Just yesterday we did not even have the concept of the wheel, but today we are exploring the outer reaches of our galaxy. We are in the midst of magic, mystery, adventure, and excitement such as Homer never dreamed of, and there seems to be no limit to our potential. With each passing moment, we make new discoveries, invent new technologies, evolve new concepts, which we then translate into action and material advancement. There is one area, however, to which we have not yet directed our conscious attention, and that area is ourselves. That must be the next step. When we begin to direct some degree of controlled attention to our own evolution, we will see the emergence of superman.

There is only one real, but significant, difference between man and superman. Man, despite his advanced state of evolution, is an entirely mechanical creature. His actions and reactions are entirely predictable. In that sense, he is no different from any mechanical device where you have an expected response when you apply a known stimulus. If you want proof of this, just observe yourself for a while. You will notice how mechanically you behave. You will realize that you are in fact "a bundle of conditioned reflexes constantly being triggered by people and circumstances." We could, in fact, take some of the most advanced intellects of our time, people we think of as highly evolved, and prove the same thing of them. Disagree with them, and notice how upset they become. Praise them, and see how happy they are. Deride, ridicule, or criticize them, and notice how depressed, angry, and hostile they turn. Eulogize, and expound their achievements and philosophies, and see them swell with pride.

The giant step that transforms man to superman is the consciousness, all of the time, of this mechanical nature of man. This consciousness gives superman the ability to control and direct his own evolution and subsequently his own environment. With this consciousness also comes the ability to transcend this mechanical nature of man, and the ability, therefore, to control and direct one's own evolution for the first time in recorded history. This ability is what the Eastern mystics and men of insight have referred to as "liberation and freedom from bondage." Our "bondage" is merely our mechanical nature.

The first step in the direction to freedom must therefore be for us to take total and complete responsibility for ourselves and our universe. Our universe is nothing but a projection of our own consciousness. Taking complete responsibility is a giant first step. It means realizing and knowing that nothing affects us but our own thoughts, that no one or no thing can ever cause us to be happy, or hurt, or angry, or frightened, or jealous, or envious, or healthy, or unhealthy. It is our own thinking, our own thoughts that make us feel those emotions. It is the lack of this realization that is responsible for all hostility, resentment, submerged anger, suppressed emotions, and psychic trauma, and in the end, all disease. Superman, armed with this knowledge, also realizes that thoughts that are repetitious, strong, and full of powerful emotion and a sense of absolute certainty are capable of transforming him and his environment in such a way that he may achieve any desired goal. Superman also knows that his thoughts are entirely under his control, and he can direct them in any manner and to any purpose that he wants.

Part III
Strategies for Healthier
and
Happier Living

The natural healing force within each one of us is the greatest force in getting well.

—Hippocrates

Chapter Twenty-one

Introduction—Self-Observation

All strategies for healthier living must revolve around the ability to change one's pattern of thinking and behavior to a positive one at all times. How can one go about this? One could make a beginning by first becoming aware of one's negative emotions by the process of what Krishnamurti calls "self-observation." One must become aware of these emotions first in order to get rid of them. Self-awareness is a necessary initial step, for only then can one try to resist or oppose the expression of a negative impulse. To quote Krishnamurti,

> It is no good trying to polish stupidity, trying to become clever. First I must know that I am stupid, that I am dull. The very awareness of my dullness is to be free of my dullness, to say, "I am a fool," not verbally, but actually say, "Well, I am a fool," then you are already watchful; you are no longer a fool. But if you resist what you are, then your dullness becomes more and more. In the world the apogee of intellect is to be very clever, very smart, very complex, very erudite, but erudition has nothing to do with intelligence. To see things as they are, in ourselves, without bringing about conflict in perceiving what we are, needs the tremendous simplicity of intelligence. I am a fool, I am a liar, I am angry, etc. I observe it, I learn about it, not relying on any authority. I do not resist it; I do not say I must be different—it is just there.

Krishnamurti's contention is that as a person begins to observe his emotions and his thoughts, and his reactions to these, this automatically results in the dissolution and destruction of negative impulses. He does not offer any technique, but suggests an ever-vigilant and attentive attitude towards one's thinking processes. It is our mechanical nature that makes us inattentive. A necessary first step in the process of becoming attentive or "conscious" is to become, in Krishnamurti's words, "attentive to our inattention." This is possible, but very difficult to do, as anyone who has ever tried to concentrate on as simple a thing as his breathing for even a short period of time will testify. However, there is a great and profound implication in Krishnamurti's advice. If it is at all possible to observe one's emotions and thoughts, then this implies a silent observer (thinker) distinct from the thought. All the great systems of meditation have sought to give us this experience of the silent self. This silent self (our true nature) is the ever present witness of our thoughts in a non-judgmental manner. Krishnamurti's advice is to constantly *be* this silent witness and in this *being* there will be freedom from anger, rage, fear, guilt, greed, intolerance, suspicion, self-pity, anxiety and depression. This is undoubtedly true, but in the absense of a technique Krishnamurti's advice is hard to follow.

In a subsequent chapter I will discuss the technique of Transcendental Meditation in detail. In my experience, this mechanical technique gives even to the beginning practitioner the experience of the silent self distinct from thoughts generated by the self. As the experience deepens and becomes more repetitive one becomes more and more aware that one (the observing self) *is* the silent witness of one's thoughts in a non-judgmental manner. This is a state of constant self-awareness (the self left alone, aware of only itself) amidst all the turmoils of "relative" existence. This unshakeable, ever present, constant silence (the self) ultimately becomes the most dominant of experiences and permeates all other experiences. This effortless, constant self-observation is a state of true liberation, for in this state no conflicts arise.

Krishnamurti: "When you attend, that is, when you give your mind, your heart, your nerves, your eyes, your ears, that is complete attention; it takes place, does it not? Total attention is that—when there is no resistance, when there is no censor, no evaluating movement, then there is attention—you have got it!"

Although I believe that true self-observation can arise only through meditative techniques, getting rid of one's negative emotions on a more superficial level is also an exciting process of self-discovery. Every time one catches oneself behaving mechanically, one gains better control and mastery over oneself. However, it is only in the complete and effortless mastery of all negative impulses that true freedom, true peace and perfect health can be found.

Chapter Twenty-two

Ego-Gratification

Believe it or not, I have several patients who enjoy being sick. In fact, I have patients who become happier as they become sicker. For example, I have a patient who, although chronically ill most of the time with a disease called ulcerative colitis, goes through cycles when she becomes acutely sick, and at times quite dangerously so. During the periods when she is chronically sick, she spends long periods of time in my office, complaining about how miserable she feels and how she can't do this or that, and how she wishes she would just die. During those periods when she is acutely and quite dangerously sick, however, she has the most quiet, relaxed, and at times quite exasperatingly carefree attitude. She may be bleeding quite profusely from the rectum, and her blood count may show profound anemia, but she insists that she feels quite normal, and despite my entreaties and her family's protestations, refuses to go into the hospital, maintaining that she will get better, and that we should not worry. When she is chronically sick, she constantly seeks attention; when acutely sick and moribund, she does not have to seek attention because she automatically gets it. The whole illness, however, revolves around the fact that the woman is constantly seeking and demanding attention and a feeling of importance.

Ego-gratification is a basic human need, and the lack of it can cause significant mental, psychological, and subsequently physical derangements. The poor woman in the above example actually becomes ill so she can gratify her ego. As a physician, I constantly see exacerbations and remissions of many disease processes according to the need for ego-gratification at that particular point in time. In other words, the genesis of disease processes can be linked to deficiencies of ego-gratification. What are these deficiencies? They usually include the following:

1. Lack of a feeling of importance.
2. Lack of appreciation.
3. Lack of love.
4. Lack of approval or encouragement.

Your ego feeds upon and needs importance, appreciation, love, approval, and encouragement, just as your body needs vitamins and minerals. A deficiency of any of these basic human needs can have disastrous results and eventually cause disease and infirmity. If we look around, we will observe that the really happy and healthy people seem to have an abundance of love, appreciation, praise, encouragement, and sense of importance, while the really unhappy, unhealthy people who hunger most for attention never seem to get it. What is the difference between these people? Is there a technique to ego-gratification? Yes, there is a technique, and knowledge of it has existed for as long as man himself. It is simply this: "Do unto others as you would have them do unto you." If you want love, pour out your love to others. If you want appreciation, praise others sincerely. If you want happiness, make others happy. If you want importance, make other people feel important and do it sincerely. If you want respect, give others your respect. If you want others to have faith and confidence in you, first put your trust in them.

There is nothing new or novel about this technique. People have known about it for ages. Everybody is familiar with some variation of the expression, "For as you sow, ye are like to reap." The problem, of course, is that knowledge about a technique is not enough. You must put the technique to use. Once you do that, you will literally be amazed at its effectiveness. It is absolutely foolproof. The technique even works at a more subtle level. Merely wishing others peace and happiness in your mind as you encounter them will bring you immeasurable peace and happiness yourself, and that ultimately is the secret of all good health and vitality.

Chapter Twenty-three

Living in the Present

Health is the thing that makes you feel that now is the best time of the year.

—Franklin Adams

Yesterday is but a dream, tomorrow is only a vision. But today well-lived makes every yesterday a dream of happiness and every tomorrow a vision of hope. Look well, therefore, to this day.

—Sanskrit saying

You may have heard the phrase, "Worry causes aging." There is tremendous truth to this statement. Everybody has seen people grow "years older in a short period of time" when they are undergoing some financial or emotional crisis. What exactly is this thing we call worry? Worry is thinking about something that has already happened in the past or about something that we anticipate will happen in the future. Worry does not occur in the present.

Let us take the former instance first. No human being has discovered a means of altering the past. Once a thing has occurred, there is absolutely no way of changing it. It is indelibly and irrevocably recorded, and there is nothing that you or anybody else can do to change the past. Thinking about and dwelling on a past mistake or a past incident is unproductive. It is also harmful. The only thing it accomplishes is to release into your system all kinds of harmful and toxic materials which raise your blood pressure and strain your heart. If you made a mistake, recognize it as such, learn from it, decide that you will not repeat that mistake, and then *leave it,* and come to the present. Know that there is nothing you can do about the past; it is gone forever, and what is done, is done. In the words of the poet, "And all our yesterdays have lighted fools/The way to dusty death."

The second kind of worrying concerns the future. Before I get into that, I must tell you an interesting story that a colleague of mine related to me. My colleague, an internist, had been treating a woman for the last twenty years. She came to see him at least twice a year for a complete physical. Every time she came, she expressed to him a great concern about having cancer. She had no symptoms of the disease, but would concoct a series of complaints so that the internist would be forced to do a series of tests merely to reassure her that she did not have cancer.

This scenario would be reenacted twice a year. Each time the internist, after completing the tests, would tell her, "You do not have cancer." And each time she would respond, "Are you sure?" This went on for twenty years or so. The last time, however, when the internist finished his tests, he had grim news. He said to her after his complete examination, "I have bad news for you; you have cancer." To which the woman replied, almost triumphantly, "I told you so! In fact I have been telling you so for the last twenty years!"

There is something about things we vividly imagine. Our subconscious mind quite automatically turns them into reality, and if we vividly imagine something we don't want to happen, which is exactly what worrying about something in the future is, it is almost certainly bound to happen. Therefore, if we must imagine the future at all, it must be an imagination of joyful, happy, and positive things.

Healthy people, however, live neither in the past nor in the future, but in the present, in the *now;* they live in eternity because eternity is nothing but an ever-successive series of *nows.* Mastering the art of enjoying your present, of experiencing as fully as possible every flavor of your perceptions as they occur, is one of the greatest secrets of health, happiness, and wisdom.

Chapter Twenty-four

Having an Open Mind

A few years ago, a patient was referred to me by a famous endocrinologist. The endocrinologist is a professor of medicine at a well-known medical school in New York and the author of several textbooks on endocrine diseases. The patient he referred to me was a close relative of his, and I was naturally very surprised when I learned her identity. Why would an authority on endocrine diseases send a patient, a relative of his, to one of his former students?

I soon discovered the reason. The woman in question had a condition called idiopathic cyclic edema. In this condition, the patient, always a woman, retains an inordinate amount of fluid in her body during certain phases of her menstrual cycle, causing weight gain, discomfort, and bloating. The cause of the condition is not known exactly, although there are a number of theories regarding its pathogenesis.

The only thing a doctor can do for it is to severely restrict salt intake and give the patient powerful diuretics. These are pills that cause fluid loss. These work to some extent, but in general the condition is resistant to treatment. The diuretics also cause loss of potassium from the body and may result in severe muscle weakness and cramps.

This patient had all the characteristics of the disease and had been particularly resistant to all forms of therapy tried so far. She would gain as much as eighteen to twenty pounds of weight during certain phases of her menstrual cycle and would become almost grotesquely bloated.

Her clothes would not fit her, she would feel ugly and depressed, and the diuretics would do nothing but cause various side effects. The patient was desperate and on the verge of a nervous breakdown. After I evaluated her, I told her quite honestly that I could do nothing for her except give her some other forms of diuretics. She willingly agreed to try them, but the new pills also were of no avail, and she continued to have all her symptoms. I wrote a letter to the professor, telling him I was unable to help her.

A few months later, I saw a very petite, slim, attractive woman at the hospital cafeteria who came up to greet me. It was my former patient, but totally unrecognizable as her former self. She looked, as she told me she had been, completely cured of her condition. She said she had gone to an acupuncturist, and after three or four treatments she had lost all the fluid and never regained the weight. She felt energetic, full of vitality, and extremely happy. I was very puzzled. How could a few needles inserted for a few minutes into different, really neurologically unconnected parts of the body, completely clear the excess fluid from this woman's body?

I took the telephone number of the acupuncturist from her and gave him a call. He seemed pleased to receive my call, and proceeded to give me a lengthy discourse on how his treatment had worked. I was very disappointed. He spoke of energy fields in various parts of the body and about how he "moved the energy from the navel to the liver, etc., etc." From my viewpoint he was totally unscientific, and seemed to be talking nonsense. I thanked him and hung up, quite puzzled. I rationalized that this woman's cure was a freak accident, or at most a placebo effect. I could not "buy" the acupuncturist's explanations. We did not even speak the same language.

Subsequently, however, I came across several other patients who had gone the traditional route in medicine without benefit, but who had dramatic benefits from acupuncture treatment. I could no longer restrain my curiosity, and decided to look once again into the mechanics of "how the thing worked." I discovered, of course, that there was a rational explanation for the effects I was seeing—that I was able to even explain some of the effects of acupuncture in my own language, that is, the scientific language of modern medicine. It was my own closed mind and built-in prejudices that had prevented me from doing so in the first place. As I decided to "open my mind" and become "innocent," I discovered a whole area of knowledge of which I had been totally ignorant. By calling it "fraud, nonsense, and stupidity" in the past, I had only succeeded in displaying my own ignorance. Unfortunately, many scientists today display a similar tendency. They are cynical and suspicious of anything which does not conform to their world view. They immediately deride and discard any opinion, philosophy, or technique that is foreign to their built-in prejudices. They are proud of their cynicism, and, in fact, believe that suspicion and cynicism are the hallmarks of a good scientist. They equate open-mindedness with gullibility.

For some time now, I have been very interested and involved in the technique of Transcendental Meditation. I have tried in vain to get a number of my scientist friends to become interested in experiencing some of the physiological effects and benefits of the technique. The very word "meditation" is enough to turn them off. They have preconceived notions of what meditation is, and they don't even want to hear about it. To them, meditation is a mystical practice indulged in only by yogis who have renounced the world and live in caves in the Himalayas. I have tried to explain to them that it is a simple, effortless mental technique that anyone can employ with profound physiological benefits, but they will not even give me a chance. Because it is "meditation," because it deals with "subjective experiences," they believe it must be unscientific, and therefore their minds remain closed to the objective physiological correlates.

A closed mind is one of the worst stumbling blocks to our evolution. It automatically closes the door to further insight into and knowledge about a new (or unknown to us) field of inquiry, and it feeds upon our own preconceived notions and prejudices. It prevents us from understanding things and people around us, and it becomes responsible ultimately for one of the greatest curses to have plagued humankind—intolerance. Intolerance is a deadly poison, and eventually it suffocates both body and mind. On the other hand, an innocent, open, inquiring mind feeds our curiosity, increases our understanding, opens up new vistas for exploration, and ultimately builds in us the great qualities of tolerance and compassion for others. An open mind is a major requisite for healthy living. It is also an attribute of the true and great scientist, the kind of scientist who often brings about a revolutionary change in thinking which finally results in a paradigm shift.

So be open to all possibilities in your mind, for only if you are open to them will you have access to them.

Chapter Twenty-five

A Vision of Wholeness and Love

Love is a creative force, and through creation one seeks joy and immortality.

—Swami Nikhilananda

The idea has been expressed that we are strands in a cosmic web. Mystics throughout the ages have visualized a thread of unity and an interrelationship among all things in the universe. The concept that we affect everything and everybody in the universe and are affected by everything and everybody has been a dominant one in at least the Eastern philosophies throughout the ages. Recently there has been the emergence among some very serious scientists of the view that the human mind may in fact be a hologram of the entire universe. This view suggests that we humans literally carry within us all the knowledge and all information that exists in the universe. The idea seems mind-boggling, but mystical insight has tended to support this viewpoint. The individual mind has been linked to a drop of water, cosmic mind to the ocean. We may think of the cosmos and ourselves as separate, but we are in fact one. The ocean is nothing but drops of water. We are like the drops of water. We tend to emphasize our differences and our individuality, but we are all parts of the cosmic ocean, and there is a fundamental oneness that connects us all.

David Bohm, a professor of theoretical physics at Burbeck College, London University, has suggested a similar world view by proposing that beneath the level of ordinary subjective experience mankind is one organism. Bohm states that, "Even if a hundred people were able to perceive the deepest stratum of reality and tap into their collective mind—the ego would vanish for these people, and they would form a single consciousness just as the parts of a highly integrated person are integrated as one." Recently Maharishi Mahesh Yogi has put forth the viewpoint that the individual psyche is part of the cosmic psyche, and that it is possible through the technique of Transcendental Meditation for the individual psyche to merge with the cosmic psyche. Obviously, for this idea to be convincing and real to anyone, the experience of being at one with the universe would be a necessary prerequisite. (We will talk more about that experience in the chapter on meditation.) However, even on an intellectual level, it is obvious that this idea has validity to it. Carl Jung had the same thought when he talked about the collective consciousness. Hindu mystics have talked about it for centuries, and modern scientists are beginning to express the same notions in their own scientific vocabulary. David Bohm uses the words "implicate order." Within this "implicate order," everything is connected with everything else in such a way that careful study of any individual element could in principle reveal detailed information about any other element in the universe.

So we are like cogs in a vast, gigantic machine, drops in an eternal, limitless sea, cells in a colossal, stupendous organism, strands in a huge cosmic web. When we affect the web, we affect ourselves. Swami Satchidananda expresses the idea very beautifully when he says,

> One day I was working in the field, and I hurt my finger. I could have ignored it, but I cleaned it and bandaged it. If I had ignored it and the finger got infected, my entire body would have suffered. The same way, if we feel we are parts of the cosmic body, the entire universe, how can we stop from loving the other parts? We are not separate from anyone; it is our duty to love and take care of our world. The head that thinks that it need not worry about infection in the thumb because the thumb is different, will get the infection itself very soon. Once you feel that you are a part of the whole, that you belong to the whole, and the whole world belongs

to you, that very feeling makes you love, and that very love brings forth healing vibrations from you. You need not even touch or see people; you just think of them. By your mere thinking you send healing vibrations. No healer can heal without that universal love. If you realize that you are not just an individual, but a part of the whole universe, you will not be afraid of anyone. A fearless man lives always, and a fearful man dies every day, every minute.

These are wonderful and inspiring words; the sentiment they convey has been expressed by every saint in every religion. Our trouble has been that while we have tended to agree with the sentiment, we have tended not to take it too seriously or too literally, and we have even tended for the most part not to put it into practical use. Scientific research is now showing that love and compassion for others is a most powerful prophylaxis against sickness and disease. To be loving and compassionate may in the end be the most self-serving and selfish thing we could do, because loving, compassionate people are in general the healthiest and strongest people.

Love is responsible for our conception, our genesis, and our birth. Love sustains us and nurtures our growth during infancy and childhood. It has been discovered that children who are emotionally deprived and suffer from lack of love have blunted and diminished levels of growth hormone in their blood. Growth hormone is a complex protein secreted by the pituitary gland and is responsible for linear growth and other very profound biochemical effects in children. This is an excellent example of the psychophysiological connection. Removing these children from the emotionally deprived environment restores the levels of growth hormone to normal and results in normal growth and development.

Love is, therefore, a powerful and primal force in the universe, and life is an expression of love and nothing else. Life may be separate from the body, but life and love are one and the same. Love has no limits, no boundaries, no expectations; it is eternal and everlasting. Love is that which gives definiteness of purpose to our lives. It is that which infuses vitality, enthusiasm, and zest into our actions. When we cease to love or to be loved (and they are the same thing), we begin to decline, and decay and death loom on the horizon.

Chapter Twenty-six

The Way of Compassion

Compassion has been defined as the sympathetic consciousness of others' distress, together with a desire to alleviate it. Compassion is mercy, sympathy, tenderness, kindness. Of all the emotions the human psyche is capable of generating, compassion is the most delicate and most rewarding. In the words of William Shakespeare—

> The quality of mercy [compassion] is not strain'd,
> It droppeth as the gentle rain from heaven
> Upon the place beneath. It is twice bless'd:
> It blesseth him that gives and him that takes.
> 'Tis mightiest in the mightiest: it becomes
> The throned monarch better than his crown;
> His sceptre shows the force of temporal power,
> The attribute to awe and majesty,
> Wherein doth sit the dread and fear of kings;
> But mercy is above this sceptred sway,
> It is enthroned in the hearts of kings,
> It is an attribute to God himself; . . .

Is compassion purely a human trait, or is it a universal quality seen in nature? Close inspection of the universe around us reveals that all life forms, from the most primitive to the most complex, display a behavior pattern that serves the ultimate good of the whole rather than the individual part. Thus, cells work not only to keep their own integrity but the integrity of tissues of which they are a part. Likewise, tissues work in concert with each other to maintain the integrity of organs, and organs in turn integrate their activities to maintain the integrity of the body as a whole. Compassion in its most elemental form is the warp and weft of the cosmic web. It is the glue which bonds the universe.

As a human trait, compassion appears as the most majestic of qualities. No process of healing can occur without compassion. No amount of technical know-how or remedial skills by themselves can effect a cure without the inherent compassion that motivates or arouses the desire to heal. Compassion heals both the healer and the healed. The flow of compassion from a physician to a patient sets into motion a complex series of biochemical reactions which ultimately effect the physiological changes that result in the cure of a disease process. Norman Cousins writes that patients are "a vast collection of emotional needs; they want reassurance; they want to be listened to; they want to feel that it makes a difference to the physician, a very big difference, whether they live or die. They want to feel they are in the physician's thoughts."

Although on a superficial level compassion might appear to be an altruistic trait, it is in the end a self-serving mechanism that restores, regenerates, and renews the person from whom the compassion originates. It would be safe to say that a deficiency of compassion is a most dangerous thing and could definitely lead to sickness and disease.

Although compassion is an inherent quality resident in the being of everything and everyone, it nevertheless needs nurture and cultivation. Buddhist lama Tarthang Tulku Rinpoche has said,

> Everything is extraordinarily inter-related. As one realizes this, each relationship becomes based on feelings of love—not calculated love, but a natural friendliness to all beings, a natural openness based on a natural understanding of inter-relationship. Gradually the whole idea of self-motivation disappears, and one sees that when you have no self-motivation or self-interest, then all your problems get solved. There no longer exists any individual problem. Of course, that is a far aim. But in terms of Buddhist psychology and therapy we can see it this way. There are all kinds of problems, a tremendous amount of suffering in the world, but the basic human problem is the same everywhere. The more I

learn of other problems, the more my own problem automatically dissolves. So it is important to observe other people's problems, not just my own, and, if I can respond compassionately to other people's suffering, communication becomes a healing link that operates in both directions. At the same time the more we understand other people, the more instantaneous and automatic is the compassionate response. All of this is the beginning of real openness. The more open you become the fewer problems you have. You are dedicated to all sentient beings, which is part of the idea of Boddhisattva (enlightenment). Knowledge of the other person increases self-knowledge; self-knowledge increases compassion; compassion increases knowledge of the other person. It is a very tight circle which can only be entered through giving up excessive pre-occupation with one's own problems.

To some extent the self-analytical schools of psychotherapy have been guilty of fostering a morbid preoccupation with one's own problems. This has resulted in a rather stunted, narrow, and warped world view that hinders self-development. Compassion shows the way out. It cleanses the doors of perception and reveals to us everything as it really is—Infinite. Compassion is the pathway to self-renewal, love, and happiness. The following poem by Rabindranath Tagore offers deep insight into the nature of compassion.

Sanyasi UPAGUPTA

Upagupta, the disciple of Buddha, lay asleep on
    the dust by the city wall of Mathura.
Lamps were all out, doors were all shut, and
    stars were all hidden by the murky sky of August.
Whose feet were those tinkling with anklets,
    touching his breast of a sudden?
He woke up startled, and the light from a woman's
    lamp fell on his forgiving eyes.
It was the dancing girl, starred with jewels,
Wearing a pale-blue mantle, drunk with the wine of her
    youth.
She lowered her lamp and saw the young face austerely
    beautiful.

"Forgive me, young ascetic," said the woman,
"Graciously come to my house.
The dusty earth is not a fit bed for you."
The young ascetic answered, "Woman,
        go on your own way;
When the time is ripe I will come to you."
Suddenly the black night showed its teeth
        in a flash of lightning,
The storm growled from the corner of the sky, and
The woman trembled in fear of some unknown danger.
A year had not yet passed.
It was the evening of a day in April in spring season.
The branches of the wayside trees were full of blossom.
Gay notes of a flute came floating in the
        warm spring air from afar.
The citizens had gone to the woods for the
        festival of flowers.
From the mid sky gazed the full moon on the
        shadows of the silent town.
The young ascetic was walking along the lonely street,
While overhead the lovesick koels* uttered from the
        mango branches their sleepless plaint.
Upagupta passed through the city gates, and
        stood at the base of the rampart.
Was that a woman lying at his feet in the
        shadow of the mango grove?
Struck with black pestilence, her body
        spotted with sores of small-pox,
She had been hurriedly removed from the town
To avoid her poisonous contagion.
The ascetic sat by her side, took her head on his knees,
And moistened her lips with water, and
        smeared her body with sandal balm.
"Who are you, merciful one?" asked the woman.
"The time, at last, has come to visit you, and
        I am here," replied the young ascetic.

*A kind of cuckoo.

Chapter Twenty-seven

Belief and Biology

Faith is the connecting link between the conscious mind of man and the great universal reservoir of infinite intelligence.

—Napoleon Hill

Although faith healers have been looked upon as frauds by the scientific community at large, recent publicity about placebos has rekindled interest in the power of faith and belief to heal. The best known use of placebos is in the treatment of pain. In this instance, the patient is given an inert substance; for example, a sugar-coated, inert pill, and told that it is a powerful pain-relieving medication. If the patient *believes* that indeed the pill is a powerful narcotic, then he obtains marked relief of his pain from this pill (which is known to have no such biological activity). This is not, however, the end of this interesting story.

If prior to being given the placebo, the patient is given a narcotic antagonist (a pharmaceutical substance such as Narcan, which blocks the effect of narcotics), then the relief of pain from the placebo does not occur. This has led biologists to conclude that the relief of pain from a placebo is brought about by the release of substances known as endogenous opiates, or endorphins. Endorphins are biologically much more powerful than synthetic narcotics, and this may explain why placebos may sometimes exert a biological effect much more powerful than even morphine or heroin. The degree of effect, or the amount of endogenous opiate release, is proportional to the extent of *belief* the user of the placebo has in its potency. So what we are seeing here is the translation of *belief* via the release of chemicals in the brain into a biological response—in this case, the belief in the placebo and its pain-relieving properties.

However, the belief could be in *anything* or *anybody* to effect *any kind* of biological response. The mechanism would be similar, although, of course, the chemicals mediating the effect would be different. All faith healing is probably mediated in similar fashion. The extent of healing or cure would again be proportional to the belief exercised by the person being healed, and in many cases also by the healer.

It is an amazing and magical thing—this state of mind we call belief. Although we are now getting some scientific insight as to how it works, the power of belief has been known to and exercised by man for centuries. The Bible states, "If thou canst believe—all things are possible to him who believes." Although scientific healing in the form of drug therapy and surgery is in our era the dominant treatment modality, the tradition of faith and religious healing has been alive through the centuries in all cultures. Even today, faith healers, Christian Scientists, and shrines such as the one at Lourdes, maintain the tradition of religious healing. Although the techniques used in these healing practices vary from culture to culture and healer to healer, the essential ingredient remains the same—belief in the efficacy of the technique, or in the powers of the healer.

A large number of New Age scientists are becoming more and more aware of belief and faith as primal forces of nature. In one sense or another, we are all believers in something. The values we embrace, the accomplishments we pursue, are all a product of our *belief system*. All *belief systems,* in turn, are in one way or another extensions of a belief system that acknowledges the existence of an all-pervasive intelligence in nature. Knowingly or unknowingly, we all participate in this belief system—even the disbelievers among us. Some scientists in their haste to be categorized as objective and astute have found a kind of snob appeal in maintaining that they do not *believe* in this concept of an all-pervasive intelligence in nature. However, the very pursuit of science presupposes and presumes an organizing power or intelligence in the workings of nature's machinery. A scientific experiment is considered valid only when it can be repeated again and again to give identical results, provided the conditions under which the experiment was performed are identical. In the absence of order, organization, or intelligence in nature, such a thing would not be possible. Thus, even the scientist who verbally professes no belief in this intelligence is obviously displaying this belief by the very act of pursuing his scientific experiment. On the level of instinct, therefore, we are all believers.

A higher level of belief occurs when we acknowledge and understand the range and nature of intelligence on an intellectual plane, and the highest level of belief occurs when we contact this intelligence on an experiential plane. It is at this highest level of belief that religious Scriptures acquire true meaning. Thus, the Bible teaches, "Thou shalt decree a thing, and it shall be established unto thee. And light shall shine upon thy ways." And again, "Ask and it shall be given unto you; seek and ye shall find; knock and it shall be open unto you." For the person who truly *believes* these statements, there can be no failure, no suffering, no ill health, no misery. Such a person can only experience strength, peace, vitality, wholeness. In the words of Napoleon Hill, belief in cosmic intelligence "restores health where all else fails, in open defiance of all the rules of modern science. It heals the wounds of sorrow and disappointment regardless of their cause, and it transcends all human experience, all education, and all knowledge available to mankind."

Chapter Twenty-eight

Curiosity and Enthusiasm

Who are we? Where do we come from? Somewhere in a Vedic text it says, "We are food transfused with thought and intelligence." We are the substance of this earth and this universe. We have oftentimes interpreted scriptural text in a metaphorical or figurative sense, but if ever there was a sentence that was absolutely and literally true, it was, "And the Lord God made man from the dust of the ground and breathed into his nostrils the breath of life, and man became a living soul."

As matter, we have always existed. The carbon, hydrogen, oxygen, and nitrogen atoms that make up our material body have always been and will always be. They were there in the primordial nebula before the Big Bang, and they will continue to exist always and forever. Our bodies have always existed as those atoms and the subatomic particles that constitute them. The print that you behold before your eyes is nothing but carbon atoms. Their location in space and time may give them different appearances, but they are the same carbon atoms that are perceived as diamonds in a necklace, as pieces of coal in a furnace, as ink in a pen, as bones in a fossil, or as the genetic code in a DNA molecule.

This is what the Hindu mystic refers to as *maya*—the universe of appearances, of different shapes and forms. Behind all these appearances, shapes, and forms, the reality is the same—all matter is atoms, all atoms are subatomic particles, and all subatomic particles may be just waves or perturbations of a field. The fact that I am here and now just happens to be an instant in the space-time continuum where a group of atoms took up certain positions, interacted with other atoms in the space-time continuum, and generated a glob of protoplasm, me. That glob of protoplasm was given a name, acquired some unique characteristics through osmosis and contact with other globs of protoplasm in the environment, and now sits at a desk writing a book.

So I am here and now, and I cannot cease to wonder what gave me, this glob of protoplasm, the capability to wonder about wonder itself. That wonderment and that curiosity are essential components of what is called the Divine Discontent, from which have sprung all the technological revolutions from the discovery of the wheel to the ability to explore distant planetary systems. The Divine Discontent expresses itself in us as simple curiosity. Look at any child and you will be struck by his or her infinite curiosity about anything and everything about him or her. The years of childhood are characteristically years of growth and development. They are also characteristically years of curiosity, enthusiasm, and innocence. The two almost seem to parallel each other. We often notice that following the turbulence of adolescence when the child "matures" into a so-called adult, he also begins to lose his enthusiasm, his curiosity, and his innocence. Along with this we also notice a subtle creeping in of a placid dullness and cynicism. Notice how this parallels the stoppage of intellectual growth, and at the same time the appearance of signs and symptoms of disease. Quite honestly, how many children do we know who complain of fatigue, insomnia, headache, boredom, or depression?

The classical academic psychologists have given credibility to the notion that development ceases after adolescence; thus, Piagetian developmental theory does not support the viewpoint that development and unfoldment of potential can continue beyond the "growing years." Fortunately, however, a paradigm shift seems to be occurring, and there are a growing number of "self-actualizing" schools of thought that are promoting the viewpoint that there is no end to growth and development, and that evolution is an ongoing, eternal process. Curiosity and enthusiasm are essential ingredients of this evolutionary process, and if we want to remain healthy and young, we must never cease to be curious, never cease to inquire into the nature of things, never thwart our own or other peoples' enthusiasm about new ideas, new things, and new accomplishments.

Chapter Twenty-nine

The Importance of Job Satisfaction

Work should be performed in the spirit of worship.
—Napoleon Hill

Various are our acts, various are the occupations of men. The carpenter desires timber, the physician disease, the Brahman a worshipper who effuses soma.

—Rig Veda

In numerous studies at various medical centers, one fact seems to stand out. People with job satisfaction have longer, healthier lives. We spend at least one-third of our lifetime on this planet practicing our chosen vocation in life. If we are unhappy with what we do during this time, it is bound to carry over into our nonworking hours. It is, therefore, bound to make us unhappy all the time, and we know that unhappiness leads to ill health and physical deterioration.

Time after time I see patients in my office whose medical problems I can directly relate to a dissatisfaction with their jobs. They just hate what they are doing, and spend their working hours filled with hostility, resentment, and unhappiness, accomplishing little in their work or their lives. After working hours, they spend their time brooding over their job dissatisfaction, and they express their frustrations in smoking, drinking, and overeating. Even their sleeping hours, which should be a time for rejuvenation and renewal, are disturbed by their constant worrying and their incessant preoccupation with their job dissatisfaction. They wear haggard and tired expressions on their faces; they suffer from such ailments as migraine headaches, heart palpitations, insomnia, obesity, and hypertension; and they look and are biologically much older than their chronological ages.

It is my experience that patients who have recently been laid off or are currently unemployed have the greatest number of complaints relating to almost every bodily system. Initially, it was my impression that these patients were people who complained more than my other, more hard-working patients. However, over the years, I have learned that people without jobs, or people who are unhappy with their jobs, actually do get sick more frequently and have more major illnesses than those people who are very busy and very happy with their work.

If you look around and observe nature in its infinite display of intelligence and practicality, one fact seems obvious. Nature has no use for that which is useless. There is nothing in nature that does not serve a useful function. The moment something stops serving a useful function, the moment it ceases to contribute to the overall growth and progress and development of which it is a part, that moment it begins to deteriorate, to decay, to become defunct, and to die out.

There is a well-known phenomenon in physiology called disuse atrophy. Physiotherapists and exercise physiologists are very familiar with it. A limb or any member of the body that is not in use will soon atrophy and become lifeless. On reversing the process, that is, making the limb useful or functional, there is return of function, return of blood flow, return of life, and the more the extremity is put to serve a useful function, the stronger and more powerful it becomes. There are no free riders, no idlers in nature. Herein lies one of the greatest secrets of good health and longevity. Emerson stated it beautifully when he said, "People do not grow old; when they cease to grow, they become old."

So here in a nutshell is one of the greatest keys to perfect health and long life. Feel and be useful. Contribute to the growth and prosperity of that which you are a part of. Very often people who hear this advice come to think they may be in the wrong profession. This may be so; however, in many instances this is not the case. It may be only that they have a negative attitude about what they are doing. One very important fact to bear in mind is that there is no job in the world that is useless. By its very definition, it must serve some useful function; otherwise it would not exist. Therefore, no matter what you are doing, realize that you are serving some useful purpose, and by doing whatever you are doing better, by contributing to the growth and evolution of that of which you are a part, you contribute to your own growth and evolution. And as long as you continue to grow and evolve, as long as you continue to develop, you will never become unhealthy, or deteriorate, or decay. If you do truly feel, however, that you are in the wrong field, that you would rather be doing something else, ask yourself what it is, and then do it. Do not worry or think about financial security or other types of security. Once you find your niche in life, your chosen career, nature will organize the rest for you. Financial security can only come if you are doing something well, and you cannot do something really well unless you love what you are doing.

One final word: beware of the word and the concept of retirement. Retirement from what? If you really love what you are doing, and if it is contributing to your growth, evolution, and enjoyment of life, then why in the world would you want to retire? If you are not getting anything out of your work, and look upon it as drudgery, then you are already retired (tired twice over). This is the time to rest, reevaluate, rejuvenate, and then plunge back into your work with new gusto and new enthusiasm, doing the same thing perhaps, but slightly differently and with a new and positive mental attitude. If that doesn't help, maybe you need a change of job. Whatever you do, however, enjoy doing it and stay useful.

Chapter Thirty

Tapping the Unconscious Mind—
The Power of Habit Force

Wise men throughout the ages have struggled to accurately understand and define the elusive faculty of man we call "mind." There have been periods in history when scientists have considered mind to be simply the non-physical or non-material expression of the physical or material brain. Thus, the brain, which is nothing but organic matter, a few ounces of tissue lodged in the skull, has been likened to the hardware components of a computer. Somehow this tissue, with all its intricate electrical networks and biochemical relay stations, generates impulses of intelligence which we call thought; and thought, although by itself a non-tangible entity, in its manifold manifestations, the expressions of ideas, gives rise to material creation.

However, the notion that mind is a function of the brain is really only an assumption with no concrete or solid evidence to back it up. Many thoughtful, well-respected scientists in recent years have offered the suggestion that mind may not be "localizable" at all, and that the central nervous system, in fact, may be just a more sensitive reflector, or "receiving station," and a transducer of a universal, non-localized field, a non-material mind. There has been a recent accumulation of clinical data that shows that damage to brain cells, or even removal of large portions of the brain, does not necessarily cause loss of memory or aberration of thinking, that any loss that may occur transiently is fully recoverable.

Obviously, there is a mind-brain relationship, but the assumption that brain is the source of mind may have been an inaccurate one. J. Lhermitte, a pioneer researcher in this field, writes: "Localizing essentially consists of placing a thing in space, and though it may be legitimate to do so for a structure or lesion, it is vanity to try to do this for a function, and it would be a great absurdity to try to imprison in a form this winged and fleeting thing that is mind."

Throughout history people have tried to measure mental function or mental potential, and this has been just about impossible. Inescapably, people have come to the conclusion that the potential of the mind is limitless, that the only limitations the mind has are those that we impose upon it. It is this limitless potential of mind that has propelled us from the Stone Age to our present era of technological wonders. Only yesterday we were struggling in the darkness of ignorance, and in a few millennia we are already on the threshold of new discoveries, looking beyond the seas of space, where lie new raw materials for the imagination. Mystery, magic, and adventure await us, and bear the promise of an age such as Homer never dreamed of. In a few millennia, we have evolved from a lowly unicellular organism to our present philosophical stature, where we ponder over the nature and source of thought and intelligence, and occasionally are even audacious enough to deny the existence of the Infinite Intelligence that gave direction to this evolutionary process. Although we are unable to comprehend the potential of mind, or even define the nature of thought itself, or devise a mechanical means of measuring mental function or potential, we arrogantly *assume* that mind may be a mechanical or biochemical phenomenon. Henri Bergson, a very perceptive philosopher, believed that "it is a chimerical enterprise to seek to localize past, or even present perception in the brain; they are not in it, it is the brain that is in them."

In order to understand the nature and function of the mind, it is convenient to divide the mind into the following three divisions. (It is important to state that the mind itself has no divisions or rigid compartments, but we create them as we create all other divisions for purposes of convenience, proper understanding, and practical usage.)

1. Conscious mind. This portion of the mind functions when one is awake. It is the mind that analyzes, reasons, and controls voluntary actions. By having mastery and control over this aspect of mind, one

116

can truly become the "master of one's fate and captain of one's soul." One can develop and refine this aspect of mind by developing more self-awareness. I have dealt with this extensively in the section on self-observation. Conscious mind, although extremely important to our self-development, our health, and our life, forms only a small percentage of our total consciousness, about 5 to 10 percent. Notice how most actions you perform are done unconsciously or mechanically and without conscious effort. One purpose of any self-developmental strategy would be to become more "conscious"; that is, less mechanical.

2. Supraconscious or intuitive mind. This aspect of mind is responsible for what is called "cognition." It is the mind that has been responsible for all the books of revelation in all cultures, traditions, and religions. Notice how similar the ideas of creation are in all religions. The supraconscious mind functions independently of thought processes and is responsible for extrasensory perception, direct knowing, and intuition. It can be refined and cultivated by contacting the source of thought, or pure consciousness, on a regular basis. This is accomplished very easily through the process of meditation and also by certain advanced techniques of meditation. I will deal with this subject extensively in a later chapter.

3. The unconscious mind. Ninety percent of our life is run by our unconscious mind. Carl Gustav Jung called the unconscious "the unwritten history of mankind from time unrecorded." This aspect of our mind records every thought, every feeling, and every impression during our waking or sleeping states. It is automatic, and functions like a tape recorder in that it is non-discriminating and will accept any idea or notion that is fed to it. It many ways it is like a computer in that the information fed to it is stored indelibly and is the basis for most of our actions, which, as mentioned previously, are mechanical. This aspect of our mind controls all involuntary activity and all autonomic functions in our body such as breathing, heartbeat, etc. It never stops, and is the center of all our habits.

However, we do have control over it in that we have control over the type of information that we feed to it. There is a popular phrase in computer technology: "Garbage in, garbage out." This applies to our unconscious mind also. By feeding positive thoughts to our unconscious, we can develop positive habits. The way to refine the unconscious mind is: a) through the power of suggestion; and b) through the process of repetition. Just the simple suggestion to oneself that one is good, happy, progressive, open-minded, non-critical, appreciative of others, kind, benevolent, energetic, creative; just these simple suggestions combined with the belief that these are true statements, is enough. The unconscious mind takes up these suggestions and programs all behavior and all action to fulfill these prophecies. Thus unhappy, unhealthy, hostile, aggressive, and self-destructive behavior is nothing but the outward manifestation of the programming of negative thoughts or impulses of intelligence that were fed to the unconscious at some time, mostly when the person was a child, either by parents or other people the child came in contact with.

However, the fact that a person was programmed into a particular way of thinking and behavior as a child does not mean that programming cannot be changed. All that is needed is the awareness that it can be changed, and then one simply changes it. It is as simple as that. Thus, people who have been unhappy all their lives can become happy simply by realizing that the source of all happiness or unhappiness is themselves, and that they can choose to become happier by choosing the kind of thoughts they wish to feed to their unconscious mind. It is the one and only thing in the world they have complete control over.

The second way to refine and perfect the unconscious is by the process of repetition. Let me give an example. Decide that you are going to smile every time you encounter another face. In the beginning you will be putting some effort into the process and often you will forget to do so, but persist in doing it and sooner or later the unconscious mind will get the message, and you will be smiling automatically every time you encounter someone. It will work miracles for you and also for those you encounter. Initially, conscious repetition is required, but over a short period of time the action will become automatic. This is the secret of forming all good habits; that is, initial conscious, repetitive effort, later replaced by automatic, unconscious behavior. In order to form healthy habits, it is best to inculcate them into one's behavior pattern one at a time. Thus, one could undertake to accomplish the following positive and healthy behavior patterns one at a time: smiling often; deciding to refrain from criticizing, condemning or complaining; becoming appreciative of others; talking less; giving other people importance.

Healthy habits are of paramount importance in determining our health status. At the Weimar Institute in California, a large poster entitled, "New Start—God's Natural Remedies" encodes a clue to some basic health habits:

N Nutrition
E Exercise
W Water

S Sunshine
T Temperance
A Air
R Rest
T Trust in God and Control of One's Thought Processes

Let us take each of these in turn:

Nutrition: I begin to deal with this in the next chapter.

Exercise: The human body is one piece of machinery that gets better with usage. Exercise reduces stress. Lungs of people who exercise process more oxygen with less effort, their hearts pump more blood with less effort, and in general all disease processes, particularly degenerative diseases, are seen less frequently. To get the maximum from exercise it must become a habit, something one does effortlessly and unconsciously, and something one enjoys. Many suggestions have been offered to help people overcome initial inertia and laziness and to make the effort required to start an exercise program. A wonderful way to begin is to exercise to the beat of music, or to catch the beat of your favorite music (raga, calypso, disco, or other). This theme has been responsible for the success of several workout programs, such as the "Jane Fonda Exercise Program," for example. Again, the effort involved is only initial.

Water: Our bodies are composed mostly of water. Proper hydration is essential to good health. This may seem self-evident, but many people do not drink enough water. Make a habit of drinking at least eight glasses of water every day. Start your day with at least three glasses of water before breakfast.

Sunshine: Some sunshine each day. One must adequately expose oneself to adequate amounts of sunshine daily. We need it to synthesize vitamin D. All life on earth is sustained by the sun. Whenever possible, make a habit of exposing yourself to sunlight for at least ten minutes a day. It is a natural and beneficial healing agent.

Temperance: This applies to all things in life, but particularly to food, drink, and work.

Air: Make a conscious effort, and it will soon become a habit, of breathing deeply ten times at least twice daily. We all know how much better and more refreshed we feel when we take a deep breath of fresh, pure air. Deep breathing clears the fog from our minds, helps control depression, induces better sleep, and aids in digestive processes. There are many advanced breathing exercises, yogic and non-yogic, which can be readily learned from several available books. A good book on the subject is by Swami Satchidananda, *Integral Yoga Hatha*.

Rest and Relaxation: I will deal with this extremely important topic in a later chapter.

Trust in God and Control over Our Thoughts: I have talked throughout this book about infinite intelligence, and a simple acknowledgment of that intelligence will give us willpower, self-control, and a positive attitude toward all things.

Habits, or habit-force, can truly shape our destiny. We can guide habit-force in the direction we want by tapping our unconscious mind.

Chapter Thirty-one

Diet and Destiny

Food is Brahman.
—Hindu Scriptures

*From food are born all creatures, which live upon food,
and after death return to food. Food is the chief of all things.
It is therefore said to be medicine for all diseases of the
body. Those who worship food as Brahman gain all material
objects. From food are born all beings, which being born,
grow by food. All beings feed upon food, and when they
die, food feeds upon them.*
—Taittiriya Upanishad

*Pure-dropping soma, bounteous food, welcome the gods at
our rite and overcome the demons and make us happy.*
—Rig Veda

Life begins as desire. Impulses of intelligence we call love and desire
bring about the fusion of minute amounts of genetic material to form
what we call a conceptus. We are conceived of love and desire and start
out as minute genetic material. This genetic material, although mic-
roscopically small, contains within it the entire blueprint of our destiny.
The material is the DNA, deoxyribonucleic acid, which constitutes the

raw material of the genetic code. DNA is made up of sugar and a chemical substance called nucleic acid. The sequence of certain bases (which are other chemicals on the nucleic acid) determines the information content or intelligence in the genes. So love and desire, born of intelligence, express that intelligence in the form of information in a material form, the sequence of bases on a DNA molecule.

We are, therefore, intelligence, desire, and love infused into the raw material we call food. Food transformed, given consciousness, is us. When we behold a potato or piece of grain, if we want it to become us, we eat it. The intelligence that permeates every cell of our physical body sets to work on that bit of nutrient. Nothing really happens to that nutrient except a change or shift in the configuration of the chemicals constituting the material of the nutrient until it becomes us, every cell and organ of us—eyes, nose, brain, bowel, heart, spleen, etc. When we partake of food, we are really participating, with the help of Infinite Intelligence, in the process of creation. It is one of the most awesome feats of nature, which, when fully appreciated, can only leave us with a sense of reverence for the almighty power and intelligence of Nature.

Consider this: I drink a glass of orange juice. Every single cell in my body, composed of billions and billions of cells, encounters every molecule of glucose in every bit of the orange juice that I ingested. Not only that, but every cell in my body partakes its share of that orange juice and converts it and incorporates it unto itself. The stages through which that every bit of orange juice becomes me are intricate and myriad. Just the enumeration of each fine detail of the process, as we now understand it, could fill an enormous amount of space in the libraries of the world. Just the awareness of the complexity, and at the same time the elegance with which the organizing power or intelligence that is in us transforms food into human beings, or other creatures of the earth, should bring about in us a reverence for: a) that intelligence, and b) that raw material that we call food; for it is that raw material that will soon become us—our eyes, our kidneys, our heart, our brain cells.

Let me say again that the act of eating is one of the greatest acts of creation we can participate in. We are, of course, as we think, but we are just as much how and what we eat. Eating indiscriminately, on the run, eating unconsciously, hurriedly overeating, not eating—these are all violations of the laws of nature. Innumerable illnesses can be linked to our diet and eating habits.

It is estimated that more than 90 percent of gastrointestinal cancer is nutritional in origin. Diet contributes in a large part to the hypercholesterolemia and heart disease epidemic prevalent in Western societies. Poor diet plays a major role in obesity, diabetes, and hypertension.

It is not the purpose of this chapter to go into detailed principles of diet, but to stress the fact that proper diet and proper attitude toward diet are essential and vital aspects to healthy living. I do not believe that it is necessary for us to be experts in nutrition in order for us to eat healthfully and nutritiously. In fact, I believe that industry and the advertising gimmickry that industry promotes have really done an inordinate amount of harm to us by confusing us and making us unsure about what we should and should not eat. We are constantly barraged from all sides by information on diet. There are beef industry and chicken magnates telling us about minimal protein requirements, while scientists are warning us about the carcinogenic nitrates present in processed meats. We cannot buy an item of food in the grocery store without being aware of the number of calories it contains, the percentage of minimal requirements it has of the essential vitamins and minerals, the additives it has, and the warning signals which go with it (such as, saccharin can cause cancer in mice). This constant bombardment and information overload, and often misinformation overload, has produced a generation of people who are totally confused and quite neurotic, and who feel they do not know enough about what to eat and what not to eat, or even how much to eat or not to eat. We live in an era where despite all our material and intellectual achievements, obesity and malnutrition, and all the ills that spring from them, remain the number one health problem of the world. So while we may constantly worry about one aspect of our diet (Am I taking the minimal ideal requirement of vitamin B6?), we may be eating without concern an estrogen-laced, fat-laden, nitrate-preserved piece of steak "especially bred for your table."

It is time to take a moment to pause, and reflect on this issue. How likely is it that birds in the forest might suffer from a deficiency of vitamin D? Is there is a single species of life on this earth other than man that knows anything about minimal USDA requirements for this nutrient or that one? Nature has blessed all its creatures with infinite intelligence intuitively, so that the snakes in the ground, the deer in the forest, and the birds in the trees know intuitively just what to eat and how much to eat. The only obese animals we are likely to encounter are those kept as pets or in a zoo.

Nature has blessed us with similar capabilities, but we have in part destroyed them by listening to people who tell us what to eat, what is supposed to taste good, what is good for us and what is not good for us. In this regard, the best advice I have heard comes from Dr. Wayne Dyer, who said, "First, be a good animal."

In part, of course, there is some justification for disseminating some knowledge about food, since we are no longer close to nature, no longer creatures of the forest, and no longer as close to our instincts as we should be. In the section on meditation, I will deal with the ability of meditation to revitalize our instincts so that we no longer have to depend on intellectual understanding of what is or is not good for us, and what we should or should not eat. This will be dealt with extensively in the section on "spontaneous right action." Until such time as we can depend wholly on our instincts for "spontaneous right action," we need some guidelines on what things constitute proper and good nutrition and good eating habits. With this in mind, I have prepared the following guidelines. I must warn the reader that what I offer here is only my opinion and does not necessarily have the sanction of the scientific or academic community at large, although many scientists do endorse similar viewpoints. I am convinced from my personal experience and from my clinical observations of hundreds of other people that if you follow my suggestions on diet, you will gain a vitality and vigor you have never experienced before. So, here we go.

1. Make eating a conscious act. Just prior to eating a meal, it is a good idea to take a few seconds to pause, and reflect, and be thankful for the opportunity that nature has offered us by providing us with food. The food we are about to ingest is to become our eyes, our hands, our organs, our affections, and our passions. It is only reasonable that we take a moment to acknowledge and respect this fact. Throughout the ages, in the custom and culture of every country, there has been a tradition of saying "Grace" or "Thanks." Like most traditions, this one serves a useful function. It inculcates in us an awareness or consciousness of the momentous act of creation in which we are about to take part. Just that awareness inside us is enough to quite automatically

result in our choosing the right kind of food and the amount most likely to fulfill our physiological needs at that particular time. The man who has just finished saying grace is less likely to gorge himself to sickness or overindulge in something unhealthy.

2. Eat only when hungry. We must eat only if we feel the need to eat. Nature has provided us with a sensation of "hunger." That feeling, not a particular time of day, should be our cue for eating. Of course, if we lead our lives in an organized fashion, we are likely to feel hungry at particular set times, and those, and those only, should be the periods when we eat. If we eat only when we are hungry and stop when the hunger is satisfied, we will not become obese. Animals do this quite automatically, and that is why we seldom see obese animals.

3. Take the time to eat. We must take the time to eat. This means we must sit down comfortably on a chair at a table, and during the act of eating do nothing else except eat. We must never eat in a hurry, on the move, standing, or while driving. We should keep conversation to a minimum while eating, and preferably not talk at all. Talking interferes with mastication, and we tend to swallow portions of food without properly chewing them. There is also the likelihood of swallowing large amounts of air, which interferes with the process of digestion and results in gaseous distension and eructation and abdominal discomfort.

4. Chew the food. All food should be chewed extremely well before swallowing. With many foods, the major part of digestion occurs in the mouth. By "gobbling down" food, we bypass a lot of very intricate and elaborate salivary enzymes and juices that nature has provided for proper digestion.

5. Eat slowly. For the above reason, it is important to eat slowly and not eat and drink at the same time.

These five principles, if adhered to, will go a long way toward preventing digestion-related problems.

THE CASE FOR VEGETARIANISM

I must begin by stating that I am convinced from my personal observations that a vegetarian diet is more healthful than a meat-containing diet. A vegetarian may be defined as "one who lives wholly or principally on vegetable foods, a person who on principle abstains from any form of animal food, or at least such as is obtained by the destruction of life." The dietary practice of vegetarianism includes, therefore, abstention from meat, poultry, fish, or other animal products. Most of mankind for much of human history has subsisted on near-vegetarian diets. The majority of the world's population today continues to eat vegetarian or semi-vegetarian diets for economic, ecologic, philosophic, religious, cultural, or other reasons. In a position paper on "The Vegetarian Approach to Eating," the American Dietetic Association observed "that a growing body of scientific evidence supports a positive relationship between the consumption of a plant-based diet and the prevention of certain diseases. It is recognized that this relationship has been established in the main from animal experimentation and epidemiological studies."

The following diseases have been definitely linked to meat-containing diets:

1. *Coronary artery disease.* Although the etiology of coronary artery disease is multifactorial, a growing body of evidence suggests that it is a diet-related, chronic, degenerative disease. Saturated fat and high levels of cholesterol have definitely been incriminated as associated factors in the development of atherosclerosis, or hardening of the arteries, which is a prerequisite to coronary artery disease. Saturated fat and cholesterol are primarily derived from foods of animal origin. When foods of plant origin are consumed in place of animal-derived foods, there is a significant decrease in levels of cholesterol in the blood. In several studies on vegetarian populations, such as the Seventh Day Adventists, there has been observed anywhere from a 30 to 50 percent decrease in mortality from coronary artery disease. This marked difference may be explained in part by the fact that most Seventh Day Adventists are also non-smokers. However, fatal coronary heart disease among non-vegetarian Seventh Day Adventists was three times greater than in the vegetarian Seventh Day Adventists of a similar age group.

2. *Cancer.* Dietary factors implicated in cancer include high fat intake, high intake of refined carbohydrates, retinoids and food additives, and a deficiency of fiber. For example, there is a high association of breast and colon cancer with high intake of fat, which is derived

primarily from animal foods. Lack of dietary fiber has been linked to a number of diseases, including hypertension, heart disease and diabetes mellitus, but the association is strongest with colon cancer.

3. *Obesity*. Several studies made in this country have documented that American vegetarians tend to be leaner than omnivores. As you know, obesity is related to morbidity from several diseases, including hypertension, heart disease, stroke, cancer, degenerative joint disease, diabetes, atherosclerosis, and also psychological problems.

4. *Dental caries* are less frequently seen in vegetarians.

5. *Osteoporosis*, or thinning of the bones, with resultant stress fractures of the spine, and other disabling bone-related problems, appear to be more common in omnivores. Epidemiological data indicates that long-term high protein intakes associated with meat-containing diets lead to calcium and bone loss. Vegetarians have about half the bone loss after age sixty years as that experienced by omnivores.

Based on observations such as the above, it is recommended that: a) one should abstain from or reduce intake of high-caloried, refined foods, that is, "empty calories"; b) replace meat with plant proteins from legumes, seeds, and nuts (commercial plant protein products, such as meat analogs, are not recommended); c) increase intake of whole-grain breads and cereals; d) use all varieties of fruits and vegetables; e) include a food high in vitamin C (all citrus fruits) to increase iron absorption; and f) provide increased vitamin D by exposing oneself to an adequate amount of sunlight daily, weather permitting.

Some General Suggestions

Foods to Avoid:

1. Any food that is not fresh. This includes all canned foods.
2. Anything with chemical preservatives or artificial coloring.
3. Foods containing concentrated sweets.
4. Foods that are excessively salty.
5. White flour products, bleached or unbleached, including white bread, white spaghetti, and crackers.
6. Coffee, tea, or other caffeine-containing drinks.

Foods to Eat:

1. Fresh food always. Fresh vegetables, such as squash, acorn, zucchini, cauliflower, carrots, kale, parsley, onions, mustard greens, cabbage.
2. Grains. Brown rice, millet, buckwheat, barley, rolled oats.
3. Unrefined oils. Safflower oil, corn oil, sesame oil.
4. Tofu, soybean, curd.
5. Flours. Whole wheat flour, whole wheat pastry flour, soy flour, fresh cornmeal, rye flour.
6. Sea vegetables, hiziki, wakame, etc.
7. Split peas, lentils, black beans, kidney beans, pinto beans, chick-peas.
8. Sweeteners. Honey, maple syrup, barley, malt, blackstrap molasses.
9. Breads. Oatmeal bread, whole wheat bread. Whole wheat spaghetti and noodles.

Some Suggestions on Cooking

1. Leave the leaves on, preserve the peelings.
2. Add as little cooking water as possible. The less water you use, the more vitamins and minerals you retain.
3. Never boil vegetables; steam them instead.
4. Keep vegetables as whole as possible as long as possible in the cooking process. Acid ingredients in the pot, such as tomatoes, mean more iron. Use such ingredients liberally.

It is obvious that a person who has had a particular dietary life-style cannot adopt these suggestions overnight. It is also obvious that a person who has been an omnivore all his life would find it extremely difficult to radically alter his eating habits. Such radical alteration might, in fact, be dangerous and quite stressful, and I do not recommend it. However, it should be quite easy to eat foods of animal origin which are low in fat, such as chicken or fish. Even in this case, however, I strongly feel the additives or chemicals, such as estrogen, that are fed to poultry and livestock during their breeding are potentially quite harmful. The best source of animal protein in my view is fresh ocean fish.

The following well-established guidelines may help those attempting to switch to a more natural diet.

1. Don't change your diet suddenly and drastically. Habits ingrained over a lifetime are best changed slowly, gradually, and in the least stressful manner.
2. Change slowly from refined flours to whole-grained breads and cereals.
3. Avoid cholesterol-containing foods such as eggs, cheese, and red meats.
4. Decrease intake of salt, refined sugar, and fats.
5. If you want to switch to a vegetarian diet, first eliminate shellfish and fat-laden meats such as pork, next red meat, and then slowly eliminate poultry and fish. Substitute plant proteins as you eliminate the meats. "Complete" plant proteins, that is, proteins which contain all essential amino acids, are available in any combination which includes whole grains with either nuts, legumes or seeds.

I would like to end this chapter on the following note. It is very important that we eat the right food because ultimately that food will become us. However, it is even more important that we have the right attitude toward food because the right attitude will automatically influence us in the right choice of food.

Regard every morsel of food as an expression of infinite energy, infinite intelligence, infinite creativity, infinite love, infinite goodness, and gradually every fiber of your being will begin to radiate those qualities.

Part IV
Toward a Higher
Reality—Meditation and
Metamorphosis

Chapter Thirty-two

The Technique—
Introduction to Transcendence

Within you there is a stillness and a sanctuary to which you can retreat at any time and be yourself.
— Herman Hesse, *Siddhartha*

Be still and know that I am God.
— Psalms 46:10

The next section of this book is, in my opinion, the most important. It is based on certain events that occurred in my life in the autumn of 1980; events that rapidly and drastically changed my world view.

I first read a book about and then had the experience of Transcendental Meditation. I picked up the book at a sale at Barnes & Noble in downtown Boston. The book was by Jack Forem (whom I subsequently came to know as a good friend). It was interesting and tantalizing in that it offered through a mental technique the experience of transcendence. The term "transcendence" had always fascinated me, but it had been an abstract word for me with no connotation of concrete experience. I had read descriptions of mystical experience, but nowhere had I come across anything that said such experience was easy to obtain or that a mental technique was readily available, so that anybody with an intact nervous system could enjoy with some simple instructions the kind of peak experiences that Abraham Maslow had talked about and that had given inspiration to the poetry of Tennyson and the writings of Emerson and Thoreau.

Intrigued, I went to the local TM center at 33 Garden Street in Cambridge, Massachusetts.* It was in the introductory lecture that I learned that some of my concepts of meditation had been quite erroneous. For example, I had always thought that meditation had something to do with concentration or with controlling the mind. I had assumed that it was meant for only a few select individuals of specialized lifestyle, and especially the reclusive, the religious, or the passive mystic, withdrawn from society. I had believed it was difficult and that probably few could ever succeed at it, even after years of practice. Words like "enlightenment" had tended to turn me off, and I had the notion that such a state was literally one of "self-hallucination," and had no relevance to the values of daily living or social progress.

Instead, I was told that: 1) the TM technique was easy to learn and to practice; that, in fact, effortlessness was the very key to its effectiveness; 2) it was an internal technology based on a highly intrinsic tendency of the human nervous system—the tendency to "transcend"; 3) learning the technique did not require the acceptance of any particular philosophical system or religious belief; and, 4) through the practice of this mental technique, one could "expand one's consciousness," and that consciousness was now becoming a legitimate subject for serious scientific study.

I must confess that I did not entirely buy everything I heard at the introductory lecture, but the instructor appeared to be a very honest, straightforward, intelligent person who believed completely in the technique he was describing, and I decided to learn the technique.

At this point the reader is probably asking, "What exactly is TM?" and I should define it. TM, or Transcendental Meditation, is a mental technique that allows the mind to experience subtle and more subtle levels of the thinking process until the mind experiences the most subtle level of thought and then transcends even that and experiences the source of thought, which is also called "pure consciousness." To practice the technique, the subject sits with eyes closed and begins to use the thinking process, with the mantra as a medium, in the precise but restful way that has been taught. Subjectively, the meditator reports an immediate sense of bodily quiet and relaxation along with "a settling down of thought activity." Often there is a loss of bodily sensation, yet full conscious awareness is maintained, and in fact is reported to be experienced as "expanded or clarified." At certain moments in the period of the TM technique, there may occur short or longer intervals where thought activity is reported to cease completely, and the mind experiences conscious awareness alone; that is, without thought content. This condition, which is difficult to imagine or describe precisely because it is a novel mode of consciousness, is the state given the name "pure consciousness." It is the fourth state of human consciousness. (The familiar three are sleeping, dreaming, and waking.)

Poets and philosophers have accidentally stumbled on this state and then struggled for years to recapture the experience. The experience itself has been the major inspiration for all their creative writing. To quote an ancient text, the *Mandukya Upanishad,* as translated by Alistair Shearer and Peter Russell:

> The fourth, say the wise, is the pure Self alone.
> Dwelling in the heart of all,
> > it is the lord of all,
> > the seer of all,
> > the source and goal of all.
> It is not outer awareness,
> It is not inner awareness,
> Nor is it a suspension of awareness.
> It is not knowing,
> It is not unknowing,
> Nor is it knowingness itself.
> It can neither be seen nor understood,
> It cannot be given boundaries.
> It is ineffable and beyond thought.
> It is indefinable.
> It is known only through becoming it.
> It is the end of all activity,
> > silent and unchanging,
> > the supreme good,
> > one without a second.
> It is the real Self.
> It, above all, should be known.

It amazed me that I experienced the state of pure consciousness the first time I practiced the TM technique. Afterwards I understood why the instructor had used terms that had seemed so extravagant: *bliss consciousness, ecstasy,* and *joyful oceanic feeling.* I realized for the first time that experience of *cosmic mind, God,* and *the Absolute* all meant the same thing, and that pure consciousness was the master key that would unlock the door to health and happiness. I knew how easy it would be to contact this source of thought on a regular basis, and knowing that gave me great pleasure.

At this point I would like to say that obviously the TM technique is not the only way to experience transcendence. Throughout history people have described unitive peak experiences. These mystical experiences are at the core of all religious feeling and tradition, and the meditative techniques and the tradition of prayer in all religions of the world aim at producing the experience of transcendence. I do believe, however, and perhaps because I am not so familiar with other techniques, that the TM technique is the simplest, easiest and most mechanical means of experiencing transcendence. In any case, by whatever means it is experienced, transcendence is definitely the master key to perfect health, sustained youth, and the easy fulfillment of all desire.

Is the fourth state of consciousness described in the preceding section merely a subjective experience, or does it have objective, reproducible, and distinctive physiological correlates? In 1971 a physiologist named Dr. Keith Wallace, then at the School of Medicine at U.C.L.A., published a landmark study in the *American Journal of Physiology* entitled "A Wakeful Hypometabolic State." He studied thirty-six subjects while they practiced the technique of Transcendental Meditation.

The subjects showed respiratory changes consisting of decreased oxygen consumption, carbon dioxide elimination, respiratory rate and minute ventilation (the volume of air breathed during a minute). Despite the marked decrease in breathing rate, the level of lactate in the blood decreased. Lactate is an end product of metabolism in the blood and goes up after increased activity, exercise, and stress, and when metabolism is increased. During the technique, skin resistance increased markedly. Increased skin resistance is a sign of deep relaxation. Dr. Wallace also showed that despite marked reduction in breathing rate, the arterial po2, or the partial pressure of oxygen in the blood, remained the same. This suggested to him that each cell in the body of these meditators was participating in the state of very deep rest, and therefore required less oxygen.

Dr. Wallace also demonstrated that during meditation there were specific changes in the EEG; that is, the brain waves. There was an increase in the intensity of slow alpha waves and occasional theta activity. There was also increased brain wave coherence; that is, increased synchrony of brain waves between the two hemispheres of the brain.

Dr. Wallace concluded that the physiological changes during meditation differed from those during sleep, hypnosis and auto-suggestion, and characterized a wakeful hypometabolic state, or a unique fourth state of consciousness. Since then literally hundreds of studies have been published in numerous scientific journals, documenting not only the uniqueness of the state of transcendence, but its innumerable benefits. A full discussion of these would be beyond the scope of this book, and the reader is referred to the massive volumes called "Scientific Research on the Transcendental Meditation Program: Collected Papers," published by Maharishi European Research University Press.

Some of the most striking longitudinal improvements noted to occur in human subjects repeatedly experiencing "pure consciousness" or transcendence include reduction in hypertension and hypercholesterolemia and spontaneous reduction in cigarette smoking, alcohol consumption, and use of non-prescription drugs. Changes in physical function have included enhanced perceptual ability, faster reaction time, changes in brainstem auditory-evoked potentials (a measure of increased hearing ability), and improvement in lung function. Changes in mental function have revealed an increase in intelligence as measured by some standard tests such as the differential aptitude test, figural reasoning subtest, and so on.

Meditators also performed better on tests of memory function, both short-term and long-term memory, and displayed increased learning ability, increased speed in solving problems accurately, increased orderliness of thinking, improved academic performance, increased productivity, better job performance, increased job satisfaction, and better relationships with co-workers. They also showed better psychological adaptability, increased emotional stability, decreased anxiety, decreased

137

depression, reduced neuroticism, a stronger intellect, increased ability of attention, increased inner control, increased self-confidence, stabilization of organized memory, increased individuality, increased self-actualization, and increased self-esteem. These remarkable changes documented in over seven hundred published studies are of immense significance.

Throughout this book, I have emphasized the close relationship of mental to physical health. A study by George E. Vaillant published in the *New England Journal of Medicine* in 1979 showed the natural history of psychological health. The study involved 204 men who were selected for the research four decades ago. For forty years, they were studied biannually. 188 men remained in the study and in good health until 1964, when the mean age of the group was about 42. Over the next 11 years, 100 of these men remained in excellent physical health, 54 acquired minor problems, and 31 became seriously ill or died. Of the 59 men with the best mental health assessments from age 21–46, only two became chronically ill or died by the age of 53. Of the 48 men with the worst mental health assessments from age 21–46, 18 became chronically ill or died. The relationship between previous mental health and subsequent physical health remained statistically significant when the effects of alcohol, tobacco use, obesity, and longevity of ancestors were excluded. The author concluded that "good mental health retarded mid-life deterioration in physical health."

Since the experience of transcendence, or pure consciousness, seems to improve mental health, a group of scientists decided to study the effects of Transcendental Meditation and an advanced version of the TM technique, known as the TM-Sidhi Program, on the aging process. Their landmark study was published in the *International Journal of Neuroscience* in 1982. In the study the authors, Robert Keith Wallace, Michael Dillbeck, Elijah Jacob, and Beth Harrington, gave a standardized test of biological aging, utilizing hearing ability, near-point vision, and blood pressure, to a cross section of people: some had been practicing TM less than five years, some more than five years, and there was a control group.

Those who had practiced TM less than five years had aging reversals averaging five years. Someone sixty, in other words, gains the health of someone fifty-five if he meditates.

However, the people who meditated more than five years actually had aging reversals averaging twelve years. That is, someone sixty who had been meditating this long would have the health, the "biological age," of someone forty-eight!

The authors concluded that together with numerous physiological and psychological studies conducted on the TM and TM-Sidhi programs, this study suggests that meditation may affect certain neural mechanisms, which in turn influence age-correlated physiological variables. In fact, it is a truly mind-boggling study of the mind, the full impact of which has not yet been appreciated. (It may be that the TM technique resets the biological clock thought to be present in the brain.)

*TM centers are located in most major cities in the United States and in many other countries.

Chapter Thirty-three

Higher States of Consciousness, Spontaneous Right Action, and All Possibilities

One conclusion was forced upon my mind at that time, and my impression of its truth has ever since remained unshaken. It is that our normal waking consciousness, rational consciousness as we call it, is but one special type of consciousness, whilst all about it, parted from it by the filmiest of screens, there lie potential forms of consciousness entirely different. We may go through life without suspecting their existence; but apply the requisite stimulus, and at a touch they are there in all their completeness, definite types of mentality which probably somewhere have their field of application and adaptation. No account of the universe in its totality can be final which leaves these other forms of consciousness quite disregarded.

—William James, *The Varieties of Religious Experience*

What is it about the experience of transcendence that causes the profound changes mentioned in the previous chapter?

Mystics and holy men, saints and sages throughout history have proclaimed that contact with transcendental consciousness is the same thing as contact with the source of all creation. More recently, Maharishi

Mahesh Yogi, an Indian scholar, has called transcendental consciousness the source of thought. Lawrence Domash, an eminent physicist, has hinted at the possible connection between "pure consciousness" and the quantum field vacuum state. To quote him,

> The pure consciousness state as experienced subjectively, and as described in ancient sources, is "eternal," "unbounded," "universal," and the "source of perfect order." At a more interesting level, the quantum vacuum state may be said to be empty (of excitation) and yet full in the sense of potentiality; it contains virtual (unphysical) representatives of all possible modes of matter and excitation in the form of vacuum fluctuations or "virtual particles." Thus, the silent empty vacuum is nonetheless lively with fluctuations of the field, which, in turn, are the necessary impulses for any "spontaneous change in nature," such as the emission of light by an atom. Likewise, the pure consciousness state is described as "perfectly silent" and beyond "change," yet is said to contain "impulses of intelligence which are beyond manifest aspects of all that can exist" and which act as the "source of all change," "the source of all creativity" containing "all possibilities."

What this scientist and several other scientists are proclaiming in highly technical language is indeed that "consciousness," the "source of thought," is "the ground-state from which all creation, including all matter, emerges." Since creation is characterized by evolution—the universe, all organs are continuously evolving, changing and improving for the better—it only makes sense that repeated exposure to this ground-state of all creation should cause evolutionary changes. From this has emerged the concept of what Maharishi Mahesh Yogi called "spontaneous right action." This whole book has developed the relationship of mind to body, thought to physiology, and has, in fact, devoted a large section to strategies for healthier living. According to Maharishi Mahesh Yogi, such strategies are really not necessary for the "enlightened individual," for he spontaneously acts "in accord with the laws of nature." Thus, the "enlightened individual," with constant exposure to the "transcendent," the source of all creation, spontaneously acts and behaves in a manner whereby "no violation of any law of nature occurs." His thoughts and actions, including diet and behavior, are always self-evolutionary. His intuition supplies him with the right set of instructions.

Let us examine a few examples of this principle. Intuitively, we have always known that smoking was bad for health. We did not have to wait for a multimillion dollar study and statement from the Surgeon General that "Smoking is hazardous to your health." On an intellectual level, science has always lagged behind, but in the end has always supported what wise, intuitive men have always known. Indeed, the philosopher William James first made the perceptive observation that the Establishment (the scientific intellectual community at large) goes through three stages in the acceptance of a new idea. It was his opinion that the Establishment first denies or refuses to acknowledge that a new idea exists. The second stage is when the Establishment admits to the existence of the idea, but attacks it as heresy or quackery. In the third and final stage, the Establishment claims that they, the Establishment, discovered the idea in the first place. For example, the idea that smoking is dangerous to one's health is largely credited to the scientific establishment, whereas intuitive and perceptive men have known this fact all along.

The scientific establishment is still struggling with the inability to make a definitive statement as to whether alcohol is good or bad for you. After much hedging, they will make such vague statements as "A little is okay, but too much is definitely bad," when it is quite obvious that alcohol is bad for health. Only recently has the Establishment begun to take seriously the role of diet to diseases such as atherosclerosis and cancer. Clearly, if we are to look to science alone for our guidance to happy, healthy living, we will have to wait a long, long time.

The above section has emphasized in a nutshell the most important message this book can offer, and that is—there is such a thing as "spontaneous right action," or "intuitive correct behavior," and that one can spontaneously acquire this through the practice of a technique that allows for the experience of transcendence. A completely "enlightened individual" would perform "spontaneous right action" all of the time.

HIGHER STATES OF CONSCIOUSNESS—
THE NEUROPHYSIOLOGY OF ENLIGHTENMENT

Enlightenment is cosmic software functioning in human hardware.

—Maharishi Mahesh Yogi

What, you might ask, is enlightenment, and what is meant by the term "a completely enlightened individual"? Enlightenment is a word that has until recently been steeped in the realm of abstruse mysticism. Different people at different periods in history have meant different things by "enlightenment." According to Maharishi Mahesh Yogi, enlightenment is simply the ability to act spontaneously in accord with the laws of nature. It is the realization that all our actions are the result of the working out of cosmic forces. When we have this realization on the level of experience, then we are "liberated." We realize then that we must act at all times in a way that allows the forces of nature to work themselves out through us, because any interference with these forces is a violation of natural law and can only result in disease, unhappiness, and suffering. This is an important point and reiterates what I have said before—the enlightened individual performs "spontaneous right action" or "intuitive correct behavior."

How does one gain enlightenment, and is there an objective neurophysiological correlate of this exalted state? Answers to questions such as this have, interestingly, come to us from scientists and researchers working in neurophysiological laboratories. In his development of a "science of creative intelligence," Maharishi Mahesh Yogi had defined seven states of consciousness. The first three of these are the ordinary states of consciousness, that is, sleeping, dreaming and waking, and the remaining four are the higher states of consciousness. Enlightenment consists of acting spontaneously from these higher states of consciousness. What are these higher states? Maharishi has defined these as follows: "The fourth state of consciousness is transcendental consciousness, the fifth state . . . cosmic consciousness, the sixth state . . . refined cosmic consciousness, and the seventh . . . unity consciousness." The fourth state of consciousness has been alluded to in the previous chapter and has been well documented, both on a subjective level and objectively by physiological criteria.

Cosmic Consciousness (the Fifth State of Consciousness)

Cosmic consciousness is said to occur when transcendental consciousness co-exists with the other three states of consciousness. This subjective experience is one of silence in the midst of activity, restful alertness co-existing with all other phases of activity. In this state, there is permanence of unbounded awareness. A person in this state continues to experience the cycle of waking, dreaming, and sleeping, but his physiology is so refined that he now naturally maintains self-awareness throughout the cycle of these states. This infusion of the fourth state of consciousness into waking, dreaming, and sleeping is said to occur with the passage of time in individuals who have regular access to transcendental consciousness through a technique such as Transcendental Meditation. It is important to emphasize that the process of becoming enlightened does not involve development of any new faculties of the nervous system, but rather consists of removal of deep stresses that inhibit the normal functioning of the nervous system. Through systematic neurophysiological refinement, a person on the path to enlightenment unfolds the natural capacity of his mind and body to function perfectly and coherently.

Is there any scientific evidence that such a thing is possible? There is. In 1974 Robert Keith Wallace, Ph.D., presented a paper entitled "The Neurophysiology of Enlightenment" at the Twenty-Sixth International Congress of Physiological Sciences. In his historic presentation, he stated

> Enlightenment means, in a physiological sense, maximum stability with minimum entropy. Minimum entropy in turn is defined in information theory as maximum certainty. As certainty is an aspect of knowledge, and as enlightenment has been traditionally defined as pure knowledge and can now be measured for its physiological correlates, the transcendental meditation technique and the physiological development it generates provide a connection between physiology and knowledge. [He went on to say,] The increased strength and orderliness of brain functioning generated by this technique is the basis of growth or enlightenment in the individual, which is validated by improved intellectual functioning, improved coordination between neuromuscular and

144

intellectual functioning, improved health—both prevention and cure, and the development of full creative potential. This objectively verified evidence of enrichment on all levels of the individuals through a procedure of neurophysiological refinement presents a vision of a better quality of human life rapidly evolving in our generation.

The most striking evidence for this fifth state of consciousness, or cosmic consciousness, comes from electroencephalographic data. In long-term meditators, the brain wave patterns during waking, dreaming, and sleeping appear similar to the brain wave patterns seen during transcendental consciousness in early meditators. In other words, there is a longitudinal cumulative effect—increased brain wave coherence is seen not only during meditation, but persists during the post-meditation period, and is seen to occur even during sleep and dream states. In addition, these long-term meditators showed the unusual ability to maintain alpha wave brain coherence (abundant during the TM technique) *after* the end of the technique with eyes open. Other biological changes that occur in these people are increased levels of the amino acid, phenylalanine (not seen in new meditators), lower levels of cortisol (the stress hormone), and a host of changes in the level of pituitary hormones, including thyroid-stimulating hormone, growth hormone, and prolactin.

Several years ago, I was involved in a study that showed that thyroid-stimulating hormone levels increased with the aging process. One very interesting finding in TM research is that levels of TSH decline with the continued practice of the TM technique. This is further evidence that the experience of transcendence seems to retard the aging process. Thus, we are seeing early, but very striking, experimental evidence that substantiates the existence of the fifth state of consciousness. In general terms, what appears to be happening here is a refinement of the mechanisms of sensory perception that allows the subtler values of perceived objects to come into awareness.

Maharishi's descriptions of the sixth and seventh states of consciousness are very beautiful. It is beyond the scope of this book to go into details of these even higher, but as yet not very well scientifically studied, states of consciousness. It will suffice here to quote what Maharishi has said about these states: "In the sixth state we gain the ability to perceive the finest relative on the surface of every object while maintaining unbounded awareness." In the seventh state, "Every object is perceived in its infinite value, the gulf between the knower and the object of knowing is bridged, knowledge is complete and full. There is no further development beyond this unified state because the perceiver and the object of perception have both risen to the same infinite value."

In the final section of this chapter, I would like to say a few words about an advanced technology of the mind that Maharishi Mahesh Yogi has offered in recent years. These are advanced methods of meditation known as the TM-Sidhi procedures. Initially, the TM technique was described as a means of creating a silent state of awareness, the state of least excitation of consciousness. The TM-Sidhi procedures have taken this development one step further and shown how "silence can be activated to achieve the fulfillment of desires and intentions from the silent level of the state of least excitation of consciousness, the simplest state of awareness." People instructed in these advanced techniques have quite clearly displayed certain creative capabilities "which in the past have been considered quite beyond the range of the normal human repertoire of behavior." These abilities include knowledge of objects hidden from view, awareness of past and future, fully developed feelings of friendliness and compassion, enhancement of sensory thresholds to near quantum mechanical level, and even levitation.

We are living in a momentous period in the evolution of the universe. All evolution until now pales before the evolution that is now occurring—the evolution of the human mind. To quote Jonas Salk, Nobel Laureate and developer of the polio vaccine,

> The principle of evolution that must be kept in mind is that it permeates everything. Before biological evolution, there was an antecedent pre-biological evolution; before that there was the evolution of the cosmos. After biological evolution there was metabiological evolution, the evolution of consciousness, and of consciousness of consciousness, as well as consciousness of evolution. Evolution is taking place within the human mind right now as a result of human experience, which we metabolize, which becomes incorporated into our being. Human thought and human creativity have all developed in response to human environment. Metabiological evolution involves the survival of the wisest. Wisdom is now becoming the new criteria of fitness.

In my opinion, human thought and human creativity will now steer the future course of evolution of the cosmos. Human thought and creativity may have initially developed in response to the environment, but now they have begun to shape and construct the environment, and this will eventually extend to the cosmos. Ideas will soon replace genes as the primary evolutionary force. Thus, we have come full circle—we now hold the key not only to our own destiny, but the destiny of the entire universe. The following diagram illustrates the point.

Cosmic mind → evolution of cosmos → prebiological evolution → biological evolution → metabiological evolution (term coined by Jonas Salk) → emergence of human thought and creativity → evolution of environment → evolution of cosmos.

Chapter Thirty-four

The Nature and Range of Intelligence

The range of creative intelligence is:
From smaller than the smallest to larger than the larg-
est.
From unmanifest through all manifestations to un-
manifest—unbounded,
infinite, eternal.
From Here to Here.
From "I" to "I."
From seed to seed.
From fullness to fullness.

—Maharishi Mahesh Yogi

The senses, they say, are subtle; more subtle than the senses
is mind; yet finer than mind is intellect; that which is beyond
even the intellect is "He."

—Bhagavad Gita

Every grain of sap contains the full value of the whole tree.
—Maharishi Mahesh Yogi

To see a World in a Grain of Sand
And a Heaven in a Wild Flower
Hold Infinity in the palm of your hand,
and Eternity in an hour.
—William Blake

The word "intelligence" means different things to different people. Depending on our viewpoint, intelligence could mean the ability to learn or understand, or deal with new or trying situations, the ability to apply knowledge to manipulate one's environment, to think abstractly, to organize information in a coherent manner, and to use that information to solve a problem. All of these definitions of intelligence are valid. Because we humans regard ourselves as intelligent, and because we equate intelligence most often with the ability to reason, we think of intelligence only in human terms and of mind as solely a property of the human nervous system.

But intelligence is much more than simply the ability to reason. Certainly the ability to reason and think in abstract terms is a characteristic of *human* intelligence and a measure of higher intelligence and intellectual prowess, and distinguishes the human species from lower forms of life. When we equate intelligence only with the ability to reason, however, we lose sight of the fact that intelligence in some form or other pervades the entire animate and inanimate universe. Itzhak Bentov defined consciousness as "the ability of a system to respond to a stimulus." In my opinion this would be a workable definition of intelligence at its simplest level. The level of intelligence of a system could then be determined by the *range* of responses possible when single or multiple stimuli were applied to the system. The more varied and complex and innovative the responses a system were capable of, the more "intelligent" it would be considered.

In this hierarchy of intelligence, even an atom of matter might be considered intelligent, albeit at the lower end of the totem pole. An atom is an entire system made up of various subatomic particles and responds in an organized manner to a stimulus. Stimulation of an atom, as for example, through the application of ultraviolet or electromagnetic radiation, can "excite" one or more electrons, which may "respond" by jumping into another orbit away from the nucleus. On removal of the stimulus, the electrons could drop back into their previous orbits and emit photons of a certain energy or frequency. Even at this level, we could elicit numerous responses from the system by applying different stimuli.

As we climb up the scale of matter from inanimate to animate forms, and then to more complex animate forms, and finally to the human nervous system, the number of possible responses to a stimulus

149

becomes infinite, and in the human mind we finally see the emergence of creative thought. But creative thought is nothing but a new or novel, or previously undocumented, response to a variety of stimuli. Creative intelligence (as applied to the human nervous system) is thus nothing but a measure of the complexity of the system, in that hitherto-unrecorded or brand new solutions (responses) occur when multiple stimuli are applied. The *purpose* of these responses ultimately is to promote growth and progress of the system, i.e., *evolution*.

When looked at in this manner, it is easy to perceive creative intelligence as the basis of all evolution. This intelligence, or this force, which seems to permeate the entire animate and inanimate universe, is what has given direction and purpose and meaning to the development of all forms of life, and has seen its ultimate glory in the development of the human nervous system and the limitless capacity of the human mind. Thus, to quote Charles Darwin, "In many cases the continued development of a part, for instance, the beak of a bird, or the teeth of a mammal, would not aid the species in gaining its food, or for any other object, but with man we can see no definite limit to the continued development of the brain and mental faculties, as far as advantage is concerned."

One "advantage" of this continued evolution of the human nervous system is that we can recognize "intelligence" at other levels of existence. This intelligence may be refined or primitive, but it exists nevertheless at all levels—atoms, large aggregates of atoms (inanimate and animate matter), and finally, even larger aggregates of matter that display a complex stage of organization where we recognize our own behavior—human beings. The mistake, of course, occurs when we assume that intelligence is purely a product of the intellect. It is actually quite the reverse. The intellect is a product of intelligence. Intelligence is basic. It is all-pervasive, and permeates and penetrates everything in the universe. This intelligence, difficult to define precisely, except as an impulse or force that sustains and nurtures all evolution, has characteristics or qualities that are easily recognizable in the workings of nature.

Maharishi Mahesh Yogi, expounder of the "science of creative intelligence," says: "The basic value of life, the field of pure creative intelligence, is inherent in everything, because everything exists and grows. The progressive and evolutionary qualities of creative intelligence are at the basis of all growth everywhere; they continually propel life on increasing steps of progress towards the fullness of life." Maharishi has further defined creative intelligence as orderly, purposeful, and integrative, as displaying an underlying rhythm of dynamism and restfulness, and as exhibiting infinite stability alongside infinite adaptability.

Characteristically, creative intelligence is also infinitely efficient and achieves maximum productivity, although expending minimal effort. These characteristics of creative intelligence are obvious in any display of nature. Thus, we see orderly movement of an electron around its nucleus, and the splendor of far-distant galaxies in their orderly paths of continuous motion. Maharishi Mahesh Yogi—"The galaxies do not just run about here and there at random; there is an order in creation; there is system in creation. Without the fundamental value of intelligence all this order and growth would not be found."

Biological processes and biological systems are even more perfect examples of the qualities of creative intelligence. Claude Bernard, regarded as the father of modern physiology, holds that

> there is an arrangement in the living being, a kind of regulated activity, which must never be neglected, because it is in truth the most striking characteristic of living beings. Vital phenomena possess indeed their rigorously determined physical/chemical conditions, but at the same time, they subordinate themselves and succeed one another in a pattern, and according to a law which pre-exists; they repeat themselves with order, regularity, constancy, and they harmonize in such a manner as to bring about the organization and growth of the individual animal or plant.

One could take any number of biological systems to illustrate the above point. As an endocrinologist, I am fascinated by the display of creative intelligence in the functioning of the autonomic nervous system and hormonal systems. Thus, the autonomic nervous system provides a significant part of the motor control of all heart muscle and smooth muscle, and of exocrine glands (such as the pancreas) and endocrine glands. It automatically, without conscious awareness, contributes to

151

the constancy of composition of fluids bathing the cells of the body; it serves to combat forces, acting either from within or without, which tend to cause variations in this environment. For example, all glandular structures under autonomic influence, the liver, pancreas and adrenal glands, act in concert to regulate the level of sugar in the blood. The entire endocrine system (hormonal system) is an example of infinite order, infinite adaptability and stability, and infinite organization. Each cell of a multicellular organism displays a complex set of controls with which to regulate and coordinate the activities of its several components.

Much of modern biology is concerned with the elucidation and study of these cellular control systems. These control systems show considerable *unity* in nature. Thus, for example, the mechanism of transporting glucose in a human muscle cell is exactly the same as that in a bacterial cell. One sees the underlying rhythm of dynamism and restfulness in the elegant "periodicities" of secretion of hormones. It is becoming increasingly evident that time-dependent changes in metabolic and endocrine function are of extreme importance. One sees periodicities on the order of minutes, hours, days, weeks, and months in all human metabolic phenomena, and it is becoming increasingly clear that biological rhythms are extremely important to health.

Creative intelligence seems to function similarly in all forms of life. The solution to particular evolutionary problems in comparative biology seems always to follow a unique pattern characteristic of creative intelligence. Thus the mechanism of utilization of glucose (known as Krebs' cycle) is the same in bacterial cells as in human cells. "The function of the hormone insulin spans eons of time from fish to man" (Howard Rasmussen). Although in the toadfish insulin is concerned mainly with the metabolism of amino acids, in the cow the metabolism of fatty acids, and in man the metabolism of glucose, in all three it serves the same function. That is, it serves as a storage hormone in the sense of increasing the conversion of foodstuff into some form of readily mobilizable energy-yielding material or substrate.

Integration and interrelatedness, also qualities of creative intelligence, are also obvious when one analyzes the workings of the endocrine system. For example, the entire endocrine system operates as a net, and elevation or decline in the level of one hormone results in the alteration in the levels of secretion of other hormones. These interrelated perturbations, however, all serve one purpose—to maintain the integrity and constancy of the chemistry of body fluids. When we study this infinitely-organized and elegantly-executed system of hormones, we are, in fact, studying or trying to interpret nature's design and purpose.

From the foregoing examples, and nature is full of such examples, it is quite obvious that intelligence does not reside only in our brains, but that it is the governing force in all our tissues and all our cells. Every organ in our body, every cell of every tissue, has intelligence. This same intelligence permeates our fingernails, our teeth, our intestines, our gonads, and our white and gray matter. It is the regulator of our biological clock, our secretions and excretions. It is also the river flowing toward the ocean, the bee in search of nectar, the beautiful design and subtle blend of shapes and colors on the wings of a butterfly, and the aerodynamic shape of an eagle soaring in the sky. So we see that creative intelligence is not localizable. It is here, there, and everywhere. Likewise, mind, which is the source of all creative intelligence, is not localizable. It is here, there, and everywhere, and it is the ultimate "ground" of all creation. However, all intelligence is interconnected and the same. It merely expresses itself, or manifests itself, in different locations in space and time as different things, objects, and phenomena. The source of all intelligence is pure consciousness, and access to pure consciousness is through transcendence.

Chapter Thirty-five

The Mechanics of Creation—
Physics and Metaphysics

Curving back within myself I create again and again.
—Rig Veda

Creation is a function of intelligence. On a simplistic level, this is easy to understand. If I want to write a story or a poem, I must first have the *desire* to do so; I must then *organize* my thoughts in an *orderly and coherent* manner, after which I must express these in an intelligible manner so you can understand them. It is obvious that the entire act of creation and comprehension in this example is a function of intelligence. Let us take another example—the creation of something like the Empire State Building. That structure as it stands today was first conceived in somebody's mind, following which a plan was formulated in either that person's mind or in the minds of several people, after which the execution of the plan (by several people) resulted in the concrete structure that stands today in New York City. So we can see here the end product, perhaps, not of a single intelligence arising in one mind, but of several intelligences arising from several minds—an example of what we might term collective consciousness. Collective consciousness, in this example, is the collective intelligence of several people working to one common purpose, in this case the erection of an edifice, the Empire

State Building. Often the collective consciousness builds upon, enlarges, and improves the products of collective consciousness from the past; that is, a previous generation. And that is the whole story of progress and civilization.

Thus, a thought or idea arose in the minds of the Wright brothers out of a desire to fly the skies, and we had the first product of that thought or intelligence—a plane that flew a few hundred feet. Subsequently, the collective consciousness of a whole group or groups of people who had the same desire and the same ideas refined and built up this product, and we had single-engined and double-engined, and then jet-powered planes. Today we have spaceships, intercontinental missiles, and intergalactic probes. Intelligence arising out of consciousness has *created* all this. We see quite clearly that creation is a function of intelligence, with *desire* being the essential progenitor.

What about the creation of our universe? Ever since man first appeared on the scene, he has sought an answer to this question. How is the material universe, of which we are a part, created? Because in man's experience creation has always been a function of intelligence, he has always ascribed the creation of the material universe to an intelligence. Because the universe is infinite, its origin must be an infinite intelligence. This idea has given birth to concepts of God and the Absolute in all religions. Is there validity to this?

Modern man is not satisfied with answers unless he can find their validity in science. Science is the new religion of our age. So what does science have to say about creation? The notions we have of our material universe have been radically influenced by discoveries in physics and by concepts originating in the minds of scientists such as Max Planck, Ernest Rutherford, Albert Einstein, and Werner Heisenberg.

In classical Newtonian physics, reality was composed basically of two things: solid objects and empty space. However, when Rutherford experimented with the atom with high-speed particles in a laboratory, he discovered something quite unexpected: atoms turned out to consist of vast, empty regions of space in which infinitesimally small particles or electrons revolved around an infinitesimally small nucleus or proton. Atoms are so small that we have to resort to mental illustrations to get some idea of their structures. A commonly used analogy is that if we were to increase the size of the atom to the size of the dome of St. Peter's Cathedral in Rome (the largest dome in the world), the nucleus would be only the size of a grain of salt. The rest of the atom (size of the dome) would be empty space.

Following Rutherford's experiment that matter consisted mainly of vast regions of empty space came another shock wave in the world of physics. Heisenberg and other quantum physicists claimed and proved that the basic building blocks of the atoms themselves, such as electrons, protons, neutrons, and a host of other subatomic particles, did not have the properties of other physical objects. Indeed, subatomic particles appeared to be "abstract entities." Depending on how an observer views it, the subatomic entity could display the properties of either a particle or a wave. When viewed as particles, one could imagine them as densely packed material in a small volume of space; when viewed as waves, one could imagine them as spread out over large regions of space. The basic building blocks of the material universe thus turned out to be concepts—the universe was turning out to be a construct of our minds, *literally.*

Mystics had made this point earlier when stating that "the universe is nothing but an extension of our consciousness." Max Planck's discovery towards the end of the nineteenth century sent further shock waves through our concepts of reality. He found that energy from radiation, such as heat, was emitted in the form of discrete packets of energy or quanta. Later Einstein found that all forms of energy, including light, could be propagated as either waves or quanta. Light was discovered to propagate as packets of quanta, or energy known as photons. The photons, although emitted in discontinuous quanta, were massless and traveled at the speed of light. So we saw once again this dual nature of light. particle or wave. The only determinant of whether light is a particle or wave is our viewpoint.

Heisenberg's "uncertainty principle" further illustrates the role of subjectivity in the examination of the subatomic realm. According to this principle, when we try to determine the exact velocity or position of an electron in its orbit at any given instance, we find that it is impossible to do this without altering its position and velocity. Merely the act of observing and measuring the orbit of the electron distorts it so much that we are unable to determine what orbit it is following. This has nothing to do with the sophistication of our instruments. Inherent in the act of observing the electron is the act of influencing it. In our observation of it, we have altered it. To the traditional scientist who is accustomed to perceiving a strictly objective world "out there," this is disturbing because it brings the area of subjectivity or consciousness into the world of objective science.

What is the exact nature of subatomic particles? We have said that they are abstract entities that may behave either as quanta or as waves. Language is inadequate to really describe some of the properties of subatomic particles, because language is in essence a product of our concepts. The universe turns out to have properties that are outside our usual frame of reference. In the words of physicist Michael Talbot, it is "not only queerer than we think, but it is queerer than we *can* think." Einstein was the first to propose that space is not three-dimensional, and that time is not a separate entity, but that space-time composes a four-dimensional continuum in which there is no unidirectional universal flow of time. He further proposed that space was not Euclidian, but curved, and it was this curvature of space-time that produced forces of nature, such as gravitation. The curvature of space-time is difficult to visualize because one visualizes space-time as having some material substance, which it does not. It is merely nothingness that is curved, and from this arise the basic forces of nature, which then give rise to the genesis of subatomic particles, which form the building blocks of the material universe.

In the modern physicists' view, there appear to be four basic or fundamental forces in nature. These are electromagnetism, gravitational force, and the strong and weak interactions. Perturbations in the field of electromagnetism are responsible for radio waves, light waves, microwaves, cosmic waves, chemical interactions, electrons, photons, and particle interactions. Gravity, with which we are all familiar, is the second major force in nature. Gravity holds the planets and stars in their orbits. It is the strongest force in the universe. The strong and weak interactions are forces in the nucleus of atoms that hold the nucleus together.

Recently physicists have formulated a theoretical framework that seems to unify all these four fundamental forces. This is the theory of Supergravity. The theory of Supergravity describes these four fundamental forces as being contained in seed form in one single giant "su-perparticle." This superparticle contains all the potential properties of the manifest, expressed, elementary particles, and the fundamental interactions of nature. The superparticle or superfield* transcends both space and time, and is the primordial expression of the total value of all manifest creation. Creation, in the language of physics, is a process of "symmetry-breaking" within this superparticle or superfield. In the process of

> sequential, dynamical symmetry-breaking, the supersymmetry is transformed, step by step, into its ingredient parts, the expressed symmetries of fundamental interactions of nature. The words "dynamical" and "spontaneous" refer to the way in which the symmetry-breaking is initiated—from within the supersymmetry itself by a dynamic process of self-referral, the supersymmetry transforms itself into its express parts—the fundamental laws of nature. All the knowledge of these expressions and the mode of their expressions are contained in the supersymmetry in virtual form.

The quotation, taken from an international symposium on "The Application of Modern Science to Natural Law" held at Maharishi European Research University in Switzerland, is an expression in physicists' language of the mechanics of creation. Could it be that these physicists are expressing in a different vocabulary what mystics and Vedic seers have cognized subjectively as the mechanics and structure of the universe? Could it be that the superparticle or superfield is nothing but consciousness itself? Certainly the description of consciousness by Maharishi Mahesh Yogi as "the field of all possibilities" would seem to suggest this. Maharishi has presented a precise picture of consciousness which is analagous to the description by physicists of the unified field in supergravity theory. In this picture, consciousness can be located as the ground state of all the laws of nature.

Science has come to the limit of its physical values in identifying the quality of self-referral in the ground state of all the laws of

---

*Recent descriptions in physics use the term "unified field" to describe this most fundamental of all the forces of nature.

nature. For all the laws of nature to be generated from their common source, that source must have the properties of infinite dynamism and self-referral; it must have the ability to create from within itself. These are the qualities of consciousness in its pure state, the field of unbounded awareness, transcendental consciousness.

The quality of self-referral is expressed poetically by the Vedic seer's cognition when he says, "Curving back within myself I create again and again." In Maharishi's description of creation, the "Absolute" or "pure consciousness" or "pure intelligence" or "Self" (and the physicists would call this the superparticle or superfield) could not hold Itself from knowing Itself, and, therefore, split Itself into the knower and known (object of knowledge). The continued self-sacrifice of the Absolute, a level of life that is never-changing, gave birth to the relative, the ever-changing, visible level with which we are all familiar. The relative is thus nothing but a transformation of energies, and every aspect of creation reflects this transformation.

Vedic scholars Alistair Shearer and Peter Russell put it this way: "The ancients taught that the universe is maintained by a hierarchy of energies known as devas (literally, the shining ones). These are the causal energies from which the subtle and gross worlds evolve, and are personified as numerous divine beings of Vedic mythology. The devas, although often of opposing values, are just the different aspects and subdivisions of the one and absolute causal energy."

The process of creation from consciousness by the mechanism of self-referral is described in poetic language in the *Mundaka Upanishad*. The language is different from the language of physics, but the two languages are describing an identical process.

> That which cannot be seen and is beyond thought
> which is without cause or parts,
> which neither perceives or acts,
> which is unchanging, all pervading, omnipresent,
> subtler than the subtlest,
> That is the eternal which the wise know to be
> the source of all.
> Just as a spider spins forth its thread,

and draws it in again,
The whole creation is woven from Brahman,
and unto It returns.
Just as plants are rooted in the earth,
all beings are supported by Brahman.
Just as hair grows from a person's head,
so does everything arise from Brahman.
From its own meditation Brahman expands,
From this comes the life force,
From the life force universal Mind evolves.
Mind gives birth to the essential elements,
And from these the many worlds and all their planes
    take form.
These worlds are the realms of action,
And through action comes the chance of immortality.
From Brahman,
The all-seeing, the all-knowing,
Whose meditation is infinite wisdom,
From this silent womb is born the creator,
Brahma,
who molds the swelling life force
into matter, name, and form.

And from the *Chandogya Upanishad,*

Very well, my son, in the beginning there was pure Being, one without a second. Some people, however, believe that in the beginning there was only non-Being, one without a second, and that non-Being gave us Being. But how could this be? How could Being arise from non-Being? No, my son, it was pure Being, one without a second that existed in the beginning.

Pure Being thinking to itself, "May I become many, may I take form" created light. Light, thinking to itself, "May I become many, may I take form" created the waters. And the waters thinking to themselves "May I become many, may I take form" created the earth. In this way the whole universe was born from pure Being, that Being which is the subtlest essence of everything, the supreme reality, the *self* of all that exists *that art thou.*

This ancient wisdom is the essence of the subjective cognition of mystics. It now appears to be the essence of the objective findings of modern science. Creation is indeed the unfoldment of Intelligence, Being, Self, Consciousness, or the Superfield into Its infinite varieties of expression.

We are one of those expressions. We also possess a nervous system that is capable of experiencing this Source of Creation. If we have the desire, we can be creators ourselves. All we have to do is transcend and then act from this field of all possibilities. This is the true meaning of the expression, "Man was created in the image of God."

DESIRE AS PROGENITOR

Desire is an essential ingredient in the process of creation. The Absolute had the desire to know Itself before It split into knower and known. The Wright brothers had the desire to fly before they invented the airplane. Every scientist desires to discover the truth before embarking on an experiment. We ourselves are nothing but expressions of desire. Our beginnings can be traced to desire arising in the consciousness of the minds of our parents.

If we are to become perfectly healthy and ever-youthful; if we are to have perpetual enthusiasm and a zest for life; if we are to be compassionate and loving, we must first have those desires. That is the first step. However, having those desires is not enough. We must be able to fulfill those desires. Fulfillment, happiness, success, health—all these can come only when we acquire the ability to spontaneously and effortlessly fulfill our desires; and this ability in turn can only come when we first open our minds to unbounded awareness (pure consciousness, the transcendental field, the home of all the laws of nature), and then activate this level of awareness so that every impulse of thought and desire is spontaneously in accordance with natural law.

Chapter Thirty-six

Reality—Manifest and Unmanifest

> *Reality is a symbol.*
> —Fazal Inayat-Khan

In general we tend to regard things that we can perceive with our senses as real, and things not readily available to our perception as unreal or imaginary. Not only that, we are apt to grade the degree of "realness" of an object in proportion to the number of senses it is able to stimulate. The more "solid" an object, the more "real" it appears to us. The Vedic Seers of ancient India divided the world of manifest objects into five different categories corresponding to the five different senses. All of manifest reality could be identified as belonging to one of these categories.

The subtlest reality was space *(akasha)*, which had its analogue in sound and could only be perceived by the sense of hearing. Next in appearance of tangibility was air *(vayu)*. Air, although primarily perceived by the sense of touch, has within it the property of sound. Thus, we can not only feel the wind, but we can hear its whistle through the trees. We cannot see it, and inherently it has no taste or smell. Next in the hierarchy of manifest realities was fire *(agni)*, readily perceived by us by the sense of sight, but also perceptible to us through the sense of touch and sound. Water was next, and identified most closely with the sense of taste, and finally there was the earth *(prithvi)*, identified by the sense of smell, but readily perceived by all of the other senses. The most "solid" objects are those of the "earth" category—they can be seen, touched, tasted, and smelled, and changing their location in space sets up vibrations, which are perceived as sounds. We humans are objects belonging to this "earth" category. We can be seen, felt, and tasted; we emanate characteristic odors and are capable of producing a variety of sounds. It was undoubtedly these characteristics that led ancients to exclaim, "Dust thou art, and to dust thou returnest."

Because our notions of reality are constructed at a subjective level, it is quite easy to understand why we regard some things as real and others as unreal or imagined. The most "real" things to us are ourselves. We may doubt the existence of everything else in the cosmos, but we are pretty sure of our own existence. The more characteristics an object possesses that remind us of ourselves, the more ready we are to accept its existence as valid or real. The majority of scientists do not accept the existence of anything that is not readily manifest to the senses.

Of course, the technology of science has in a way extended (and continues to extend) the range of things available to our senses. Thus, with the help of a radio receiver, we can extend our sense of hearing and pick up sounds emanating from other parts of the world, or even those coming from outer space. Without the radio set, we would have no idea that such sounds are actually around us all the time, and would feel quite justified in denying their existence. Likewise, with the television screen in front of us, we can extend our sense of sight so that we can see astronauts perform their spacewalks, or jump over craters on the surface of the moon. With the help of scientific technology, we have in fact refined our sense of sight to the extent that we can gaze through powerful telescopes at stars millions of light-years away and literally cross the time barrier to behold today what existed millions of years ago. Without this kind of technology, we would feel quite justified in denying the existence of things not readily apparent to our eyes.

It becomes obvious immediately that we "construct" reality according to our perception. The limits of our perception, however, keep continually expanding as we devise more and more sophisticated methods of enlarging our sensory abilities—be it an electron microscope, a quasar detector, or a seismograph. All perception, however, ultimately occurs in the mind. It is the mind that ultimately sees, hears, tastes,

163

touches or smells, and it is the mind ultimately that devises those instruments that augment or otherwise make readily available to perception objects ordinarily hidden to our senses. Reality in its ultimate nature is a construct of our minds—*we make reality*. It has no existence outside of our minds and our experience. The shape, size, appearance, or any other attribute of an object is a purely subjective quality.

Let us take an example. Imagine for a moment that the lens of the human eye was square or some other shape instead of its usual oval shape. Just this change in one aspect of the sensory apparatus responsible for vision would completely alter the appearance of the whole world as perceived by human eyes. A marble perceived through this different-shaped lens in the eye might appear as having the shape of a pencil. If all human beings had this different square or other-shaped lens in their eyes, we would all agree that a marble would be a different-looking object from what we now know it to be. Another species, a rabbit for example, which has rods and cones (the light perceiving receptors) arranged in a different pattern on the retina (as compared to ours), may perceive the marble as having even another shape. The question is—what is the real shape of the marble? The answer is—there is no such shape as the real shape. The marble has no shape independent of a perceiver. It is the perception that gives the marble its shape. This same phenomenon holds true for all the other senses—so that we come to the astounding conclusion that the marble has no independent existence outside of the perceiver. In other words, it would not exist were there not a mind to perceive it.

Perception itself is not only limited by the range of the senses but is shaped, even at physiological level, by previous experience. A simple experiment with kittens conducted by Helmut and Spinelli exemplifies this. Three batches of kittens were raised in three separate environments. One set of kittens was brought up in an environment that was totally horizontal (horizontal stripes). Another set of kittens grew up in a completely vertical world (vertical stripes). A third set was kept in a totally blank white area. When these kittens became adult cats they perceived the world differently from each other. The kittens exposed to a world of horizontal patterning had perfect ability to see things that were horizontal, but were unable to actually see anything that was vertical. They would bump into everything vertical—such as furniture legs, for example. The vertical stripers could see only vertical objects and were blind to everything horizontal. The kittens kept in a white area in which there was no detail failed to develop a normal adult-cat visual sense. This was not a question of belief. The brains of these cats were sensitive to only a limited aspect of the continuum of visual stimuli present in nature.

In another experiment, by Greenough, it was found that if one eye of a newborn monkey was closed for a prolonged period, the connections from both sides of the brain to the open eye increased while the connection to the closed eye decreased and finally disappeared, leading ultimately to blindness in the closed eye. This experiment corroborates the findings of the experiment with kittens in suggesting that electrical patterns activated by an animal's previous experience modulate the neuronal connections and receptors that result in perception. The very structure of the brain itself, where all perception ultimately occurs, is dependent on and influenced by our previous experiences of the world. In the words of the ancient mystic Rumi "new organs of perception come into being as a result of necessity." But perception gives us experience. We see here a very tight circle; perception shapes experience and experience shapes perception. What we have to realize, however, is that both perception and experience are *created* by the mind. The material world does not exist independently of the mind.

Stated differently, *without the mind there is no material universe*. The material world is quite literally a mirage, an ephemeral thing that the mind has created. The mind, although unmanifest by itself, displays its reality through manifest material objects. The material objects are not real, however. The only real and tangible thing is the unmanifest mind that creates them. The mind is the source; you and I are the source. Our entire reality comes from us, from our ideas, our notions. Reality is merely the symbolic manifest expression of the unmanifest idea. To create something out there, all we have to do is first agree between us that a certain reality exists out there, and that agreement between us would then construct that reality. You see, what you and I call reality is nothing but an expression of our collective consciousness. Our collective consciousness agrees that the reality exists. Before anything becomes a reality, it exists in seed form as a perturbation in the collective consciousness of society. That perturbation initially manifests itself as a vague notion, then sprouts into an idea, and finally expresses itself as reality. You and I (our collective consciousness) agree on wars, we construct wars in our minds, then we have wars. Wars are a manifestation of stress in the collective consciousness of a society. If we did not agree to have wars, wars would not exist. Right at this moment, everything that is real is what you and I, and everybody (our collective consciousness) have constructed, consciously or unconsciously, from our notion or idea of what constitutes reality. We get sick, we grow old, we become disabled because of our notions and ideas that these are realities. We were told that, we accept that, we construct those realities. So we get sick and grow old. If we did not have those notions first, we would not necessarily become those realities.

The key to our universe lies in the fact that we can choose. Before we choose, we must become aware that we generate the ideas that manifest our realities. Once we become aware of this fact, we could choose only those notions or ideas that would serve an evolutionary function. Because we have up to now chosen fear, greed, hatred, wars, disease, and death, these are our realities. We could now choose courage, love, peace, health, and immortality, and they would become our realities. We could even create the legendary fountain of youth by simply expressing in our collective consciousness the notion or idea that we can choose to be healthy and young forever. Until now our notion of age has been what "they" (the collective consciousness) have told us. That is why we are getting older. Growing old is in large measure simply a notion, an idea reflected in reality. If we are to change that reality, we have to first generate a different notion in our collective consciousness. Our bodies, our brains, are simply living expressions of our notions and ideas of our world view. We as pure consciousness are at the source: pure being, ourself, is the originator of all notions. By diving deep into our source—the source of thought, the field of pure intelligence, the field where all possibilities exist—we can create any reality we choose to construct. Perfect health, everlasting peace, even immortality, are now available to us as notions. Having those notions in our individual consciousness is a necessary first step in their expression, but only when they become deeply entrenched in our collective consciousness will they translate into living realities.

Chapter Thirty-seven

One Is All, and All Is One

A paradigm is a theoretical framework that explains a set of scientifically determined data. It is a hypothesis commonly accepted by the majority of people at a particular moment in history. Thus the observation that one sees the sun in the east in the morning and in the west in the evening could lead to two equally reasonable hypotheses: (a) the sun rises in the east and sets in the west, or (b) the sun neither rises nor sets; it is the earth spinning on its axis that gives us this optical illusion. Both hypotheses are equally valid since they both explain our initial observation. In fact, there was a time in history when the majority of people in the world believed in hypothesis (a). Until about 1543, that was the prevailing paradigm. However, when astronomers began to make observations that did not fit this theoretical framework, a new paradigm, i.e., hypothesis (b), had to be constructed. Is the second paradigm the correct one? All of us assume that it is. However, if new observations are made that cannot be explained by hypothesis (b), then we may have to develop yet another set of theories. These theories in and of themselves are neither true nor untrue. They are simply the best possible explanations at a given point in time for scientifically observed facts.

The paradigm, therefore, is not a fact in itself, but a concept. It may start off as a concept in the mind of a single person, but it does not become a paradigm until it becomes a concept commonly held by a majority of people. The fact that the concept is held by the majority of people does not make it intrinsically correct or incorrect. It merely gives it validity by common agreement. Thus a paradigm in reality is nothing but an expression of collective consciousness. It is the algebraic sum of the ideas, beliefs, prejudices, assumptions and symbols common to all mankind at a particular moment in history. It is easy to understand that the introduction of a new paradigm meets with great resistance. Its acceptance requires a change in collective consciousness, a transformation of almost the entire human psyche. This also explains why it is difficult for people to accept certain facts if they do not fit into the accepted theoretical framework, and why perfectly valid observations may be dismissed as anomalous data when in fact it is the prevailing paradigm that is anomalous.

We are currently in the throes of a paradigm shift that is challenging our mechanistic world view with very surprising and yet very testable alternatives.

Let us consider some extremely fascinating data obtained from experiments in both animals and human beings.

1. If a number of rats are trained to carry out a task which they have never performed before (such as, for example, going through a complicated maze) then according to a report in *Science Digest,* rats elsewhere in the world are able to carry out the same task much more easily. These other rats are in no way genetically related to the original rats and have no physical connection or communication with the original rats. In other words, rats in one place would come out of a maze more quickly because rats in another place had already solved the problem. How do you explain this phenomenon?

2. Even more fascinating is the story of a colony of Japanese monkeys on the island of Koshima in Japan. The story is recounted by biologist Lyall Watson in his book *Lifetide.* The monkeys on this island lived on a diet of sweet potatoes that had been dropped in the sand by scientists. The monkeys found it extremely difficult to eat these sweet potatoes because they were covered with sand and grit. However, in 1952,

> an eighteen-month-old female, a sort of monkey genius called Imo, solved the problem by carrying the potatoes down to a stream and washing them before feeding. In monkey terms this is a

cultural revolution comparable almost to the invention of the wheel.

Many other monkeys subsequently learned this trick by watching Imo and one another, and according to Watson,

> by 1958, all the juveniles were washing dirty food, but the only adults over five years old to do so were the ones who learned by direct imitation from their children.

Then something extraordinary happened.

> In the autumn of that year an unspecified number of monkeys on Koshima were washing sweet potatoes in the sea, because Imo had made the further discovery that salt water not only cleaned the food but gave it an interesting new flavor. Let us say, for argument's sake, that the number was ninety-nine and that at eleven o'clock on a Tuesday morning, one further convert was added to the fold in the usual way. But the addition of the hundredth monkey apparently carried the number across some sort of threshold, pushing it through a kind of critical mass, because by that evening almost everyone in the colony was doing it. Not only that, but the habit seems to have jumped natural barriers and to have appeared spontaneously, like glycerin crystals in sealed laboratory jars, in colonies on other islands and on the mainland in a troop at Takasakiyama.

Watson believes this anecdote has relevance because "it suggests there may be mechanisms in evolution other than those governed by natural selection." He thinks that humans have gone through a hundredth-monkey experience and that the explosive growth in the style and complexity of human culture about one hundred thousand years ago must have been a similar experience. He writes,

> I believe it was in this period that human language passed from a simple and probably highly ritualized system of sound to a true language full of complex conceptual invention—that this was the moment in time when we pulled several of the old threads together and began to build a full oral tradition. There is some evidence

169

to suggest too that it was also at this time that man progressed from simply scavenging to become a truly efficient hunter. . . . Everything points to a comparatively short period of evolutionary ferment and rapid growth and change. The most interesting feature of the changes is that they were widespread and made on all locations at almost exactly the same time. This synchronicity is as difficult to explain as the sudden outbreak of pandemics in widely separated places, long before the advent of movement and trade. Unless one assumes the existence of a common factor, perhaps even the same factor—a new set of instructions.

Watson thinks that the hundredth-monkey phenomenon might account for the way memories, ideas, and fashions spread through human culture. "It may be that when enough of us hold something to be true, it becomes true for everyone."

3. The most striking experiment of a similar nature in humans concerns the so-called "Maharishi effect." The fact that practice of the TM Program and TM-Sidhi Program improves health and cognitive and behavioral functioning has been validated in numerous scientific studies and is easy to explain on the basis of the physiological benefits derived from the technique. However, in 1976 Dr. Candace Borland, a psychologist in Switzerland, published a study that certainly challenges our notions of credibility when we first glance at it. Dr. Borland's study focused on the relationship between percentage of the population in a city practicing the TM technique in a given year and change in crime rate in the following year.

Dr. Borland discovered that when about one percent of the population of a city practiced TM, the crime rate dropped as much as 16%. (Dr. Borland's study compared eleven U.S. cities in the 25,000–50,000 population range with matched control cities.) Further analysis indicated that factors other than the cities' reaching about one percent of their populations practicing the TM technique were unlikely to account for the subsequent change in crime rate in these cities. These results, in fact, were consistent with the prediction made by Maharishi Mahesh Yogi, founder of the Transcendental Meditation Program, that when about one percent of a population practiced the TM technique a "phase transition in society toward more harmonious functioning would occur." Therefore this phenomenon was named the "Maharishi effect."

170

A subsequent study published in the *Journal of Crime and Justice* in 1981 validated Dr. Borland's study on the effect of one percent of the population in a city practicing the TM technique in a sample of forty-eight cities. Statistical procedures were employed to control for the effects of other factors that may have influenced outcomes, such as prior crime trends, police coverage, educational level, population density and stability, college education and unemployment rates. Since then nine independent studies have provided evidence that small numbers practicing the TM technique (as little as one percent of the larger population) can spontaneously reduce negative trends, not only in those with whom they directly interact, but throughout the whole society as well. The effect gets amplified when an advanced variant of the technique known as the TM-Sidhi program is practiced. During periods when there is regular collective practice of the TM-Sidhi technique by as little as one percent of the population, beneficial changes in the whole society are observed as a result of the "super-radiance" generated by the collective practice.

These findings have been predicted and replicated in at least ten separate studies on city, provincial, and national levels, in relation to social problems such as violent crime, death from civil order, accidents and suicides, strikes, air pollution, and traffic violations, and in relation to economic growth and stability and improved international relations. The studies are so impressive that an Institute for Research on Consciousness and Human Development has been established in Cambridge to "evaluate promising means for enhancing social development and resolving conflict on a national and international scale." The Institute is affiliated with the Harvard University Department of Psychology and Social Relations and is headed by Dr. Charles Alexander, a Harvard psychologist, and himself a practitioner and teacher of the TM technique.

How do we explain the above-mentioned phenomena? How do we fit them into our current paradigm? The answer is that we cannot fit them into our current conceptual scheme. We have to develop a new hypothesis to explain them. The picture we are seeing does not neatly fit into our framework. We have to change the framework.

Dr. Rupert Sheldrake, a prominent plant physiologist, has postulated the hypothesis of "formative causation" to explain some of these findings. In an article entitled "Hidden Force" published in *Science Digest* he states that "the characteristic forms taken up by molecules, crystals, cells, tissues, and organisms are shaped and maintained by specific fields called *morphogenetic fields* (from the Greek *morphe,* form, and 'genesis,' coming into being). The structure of these fields is derived from the morphogenetic fields associated with previously similar systems; the morphogenetic fields of past systems influence subsequent similar systems by a process called *morphic resonance.*" Dr. Sheldrake explains everything from the formation of crystals to the learning of new behavior by animals through the hypothesis of morphic resonance. Dr. Sheldrake does not, however, say what these fields are—what is their composition and what are they made of?

Could it be that these fields are consciousness itself? Scientists David Orme-Johnson, Michael C. Dillbeck, and Robert Keith Wallace published a paper in the *International Journal of Neuroscience* in 1982 entitled "Intersubject EEG Coherence: Is Consciousness a Field?" Coherence is a mathematical quality that provides a measure of the constancy of the relationship of different phases of the EEG (brain waves) at a specified frequency when measured at two spatially separated parts of the scalp. Increased coherence between different parts of the brain is a sign of greater orderliness in the brain, but it also is evidence of the fact that the different parts in displaying coherence with each other are displaying some kind of connection or communication with each other. Therefore, when we say that two cerebral hemispheres show increased coherence, we are in essence saying that there is increased communication between the two hemispheres of the brain. Intersubject EEG coherence would, therefore, signify that there was some kind of communication between the brains of two different subjects. It was as if the two brains were behaving as one. If there was intersubject coherence between several subjects, we would have several brains behaving as one—a sort of collective brain.

This is exactly what scientists David Orme-Johnson, Dillbeck, and Wallace showed. They measured EEG coherence *between* pairs of three different subjects during a one-hour period practice of the Transcendental Meditation program. Coherence between subjects was evaluated for two sequential fifteen-minute periods. On six experimental days, these periods preceded and then coincided with the fifteen-minute period during which 2500 students participated in the TM-Sidhi program at a course over one thousand miles away. After the course had ended, coherence was evaluated on six control days. It was found that inter-subject coherence was generally low with coherence in the alpha and beta frequencies significantly higher than at other frequencies. On the experimental days, intersubject coherence increased during the experimental period relative to the fifteen-minute baseline period immediately preceding the experimental period. Coherence increased significantly from baseline to experimental periods on experimental days compared with control days. This effect was particularly evident in the alpha and beta frequencies.

According to the authors, these results reinforced previous sociological studies showing decreased social disorder in the vicinity of TM and TM-Sidhi participants. The authors concluded their paper as follows:

> Regardless of what the conclusive theoretical explanation of the present experimental results may be, this approach points to a novel neurophysiological approach to studying the sociological effects reported to be produced by the TM and TM-Sidhi techniques, and perhaps other social phenomena as well. They indicate that this remarkable new technology for creating coherence in collective consciousness could potentially lead not only to the improvement of the quality of life in cities, as the crime studies cited above suggest, but also to the resolution of international conflicts and the establishment of world peace.

It is becoming obvious that the new paradigm we are constructing will be based on the assumption that Consciousness is the ultimate ground of all that we can hear, see, touch, taste, and smell. This idea has in essence existed since human thought first surfaced, but only now is beginning to acquire scientific validity. The notion that Consciousness manifests itself as the seeming many elements of the material world was first encountered in Hindu scriptures, and is the foundation of all Oriental philosophies, and also those of Emerson, Hegel, Leibnitz, Schopenhauer, Descartes, and Spinoza. The following statement, which I discovered in a book by Wallace D. Wattles, published in 1915, summarizes the entire message of this book.

There is a formless thinking stuff from which all things are made, and which in its original state, permeates, penetrates, and fills the interspaces of the universe.

A thought in this substance produces the thing that is imaged by the thought.

Man can form things in his thought, and, by impressing his thoughts upon formless substance, can cause the thing he thinks about to be created.

Realization of the truth of this statement, not just emotionally, not just philosophically, or intellectually, but experientially, is the master key to perfect health, happiness, and all good things in life.

Epilogue—The Future

When a major paradigm shift occurs, several things happen. First, we begin to have an understanding of what were previously (to us) inexplicable phenomena. Second, with our new insight, we develop the ability to make certain predictions about the future.

The last section of this book has focused attention on the theme that Consciousness is a field of all possibilities, and that the intellectual, but more importantly, the experiential understanding of this fact is indeed the master key to perfect health and happiness. At this time, for those of you who have come this far in your reading, I would like to recapitulate and summarize the basic principles of this new conceptual framework, following which I would like to make some predictions about the future:

1. Consciousness is Absolute. It exists. It transcends both space and time.
2. When Consciousness (the Absolute) moves within itself, it gives rise to impulses of intelligence (the Relative). In the language of physics, by a process of symmetry-breaking and self-referral, the Superfield (Consciousness) gives rise to the basic forces of nature (impulses of intelligence)—the strong and weak interactions, gravity, electromagnetism, etc.
3. Impulses of intelligence (basic forces) give rise to all material creation.
4. Material creation may be divided into subjective and objective. These may also be called perceiver and perceived (object of perception).

175

5. The interaction of subject and object (perceiver and perceived) gives rise to another sub-species of intelligence—human thought.
6. The application of human thought results in the further interaction of subject and object, giving rise to scientific achievement and technology.
7. Knowledge, which is the basic requirement for any achievement, may be objective or subjective.
8. Both objective knowledge and subjective knowledge are necessary for the full realization of a person's potential.
9. Objective knowledge leads to technical know-how; subjective knowledge results in spontaneous right action.
10. Spontaneous right action, or intuitive correct behavior, is a prerequisite for perfect health.
11. It is possible to achieve the ability to act without making mistakes (perfection) by experiencing the field of Consciousness at regular intervals.
12. The experience is available through a mechanical technique such as Transcendental Meditation.

Based on these principles, certain predictions can be made about the future:

1. More and more people will have access to an understanding of the field of Consciousness.
2. In the coming years, we will see a decline in morbidity and mortality from such now relatively common diseases as cancer, heart attacks, stroke and hypertension, and from accidents.
3. People will live longer and healthier lives. Both objective knowledge (scientific advancement) and subjective knowledge (spontaneous right action) will lead to a new breed of human beings. There will be continued life extension in the direction of immortality.
4. Clearer experience of the field of Consciousness among larger groups of people will lead to the ability by these people to activate this field (as in the Sidhis). We will see

the acceptance and the common demonstration of unusual abilities among highly developed persons. These will include fully developed feelings of friendliness and compassion, enhancement of sensory thresholds to near quantum levels, awareness of past and future, knowledge of objects hidden from view, intuition and levitation.

5. The understanding of the group dynamics of Consciousness will ultimately lead to its application (successfully) to the solving of social problems, to the enhancement of material prosperity, and finally to the development of world peace (which is the perfection of societal health).

Bibliography

BOOKS

Bentov, Itzhak. *Stalking the Wild Pendulum: On the Mechanics of Consciousness*. New York: Bantam New Age Books, 1979.

Bloomfield, Harold H., M.D., Cain, Michael Peter, Jaffe, Dennis T., and Corey, Robert P. *TM: Discovering Inner Energy and Overcoming Stress*. New York: Dell Publishing Co., Inc., 1975.

Bristol, Claude M. *The Magic of Believing*. New York: Pocket Books, 1948.

Campbell, Anthony. *TM and the Nature of Enlightenment*. New York: Harper & Row Publishers, 1975.

Choate, Burt G. *The Core of Creation: An Investigation into the Fundamentals of Reality and the Foundation of Existence*. Rush, New York: Syzygy Publications, 1982.

Cooper, J. T., M.D. *Dr. Cooper's Fabulous Fructose Diet*. New York: M. Evans & Co., 1979.

Dossey, Dr. Larry. *Space, Time and Medicine*. Boulder, Colorado: Shambhala Publications, Inc., 1982.

Durant, William. *Our Oriental Heritage*. New York: Simon and Schuster, 1954.

Dyer, Dr. Wayne. *The Sky's the Limit*. New York: Simon and Schuster Pocket Books, 1980.

Forem, Jack. *Transcendental Meditation, Maharishi Mahesh Yogi and the Science of Creative Intelligence*. New York: E. P. Dutton and Co., Inc., 1973.

Goswami, Amit. *The Cosmic Dancers*. New York: Harper & Row, 1983.

Hill, Napoleon. *Law of Success*. Chicago: Success Unlimited, Inc., 1979.

Hillman, James. *Insearch: Psychology and Religion*. New York: Charles Scribner's Sons, 1967.

Krishnamurti, J. *The Wholeness of Life*. New York: Harper & Row Publishers, 1979.

———— *You Are the World*. New York: Harper & Row Publishers, 1972.

179

Murphy, Joseph. *The Cosmic Power within You*. West Nyack, N.Y.: Parker Publishing Company, Inc. 1968.

Needleman, Jacob, and Lewis, Dennis, editors. *On the Way to Self-Knowledge*. New York: Alfred A. Knopf, 1976.

Orme-Johnson, David W., Farrow, John T., and Domash, Lawrence, editors. *Scientific Research of the Transcendental Meditation Program, Collected Papers*, Volume 1. Switzerland: MERU Press, 1976.

Pearson, Durk and Shaw, Sandy. *Life Extension*. New York: Warner Books, 1982.

Rasmussen, Howard. *Textbook of Endocrinology* (Fifth Edition). Ed. Robert H. Williams. Philadelphia: W. B. Saunders Company, 1974.

Restak, M. Richard. *The Brain—The Last Frontier*. New York: Warner Books, 1979.

Satchidananda, Swami. *Beyond Words*. New York: Holt, Rinehart, and Winston, 1977.

———. *Integral Yoga Hatha*. New York: Holt, Rinehart, and Winston, 1970.

Shearer, Alistair, and Russell, Peter, trans. *The Upanishads*. New York: Harper & Row, 1978.

Smith, Adam. *Powers of Mind*. New York: Summit Books, 1975.

Tagore, Rabindranath. *Collected Poems and Plays of Rabindranath Tagore*. New York: Macmillan, 1956.

Talbot, Michael. *Mysticism and the New Physics*. New York: Bantam New Age Books, 1981.

Van Over, Raymond. *Eastern Mysticism*. New York: New American Publishers, Mentor Books, 1977.

Vernon, Howard. *Pathways to Perfect Living*. New York: Stein & Day Publishers, 1978.

———. *The Mystic Path to Cosmic Power*. West Nyack, N.Y.: Parker Publishing Company, Inc., 1967.

Watson, Lyall. *Lifetide*. New York: Simon and Schuster, 1979.

Wattles, Wallace D. *The Science of Getting Rich*. Lakemont, Georgia: Copple House, 1975.

Weitzman, D. Eliot, editor. *Advances in Sleep Research*, Volume 1. Flushing, N.Y.: Spectrum Publications, Inc., 1974.

Wood, E. Ernest. *The Glorious Presence*. Wheaton, Illinois: The Theosophical Publishing House, 1951.

Yogi, Maharishi Mahesh. *Bhagavad Gita, A New Translation and Commentary*. Chapters 1–6. New York: Penguin Books, 1969.

———. *The Science of Being and the Art of Living*. New York: MIU Press, Livingston Manor, 1963.

Zukav, Gary. *The Dancing Wu Li Masters, an Overview of the New Physics*. New York: Bantam New Age Books, 1979.

PERIODICALS AND PROCEEDINGS

"The Application of Modern Science and Natural Law," *Proceedings of the International Symposium*. Seelisberg, Switzerland: Maharishi European Research University, March 12–14, 1982.

Baum, David and John Wellwood. "Issues in Physics, Psychology and Metaphysics." *Journal of Transpersonal Psychology*, Volume 12, No. 1 (1980).

"Diet, Nutrition and Cancer." *Cancer Research*. The National Research Council, Volumes 43–46 (June 1983), pp. 3018–3023.

Greenough, W. "Development and Memory: The Synaptic Connection," *Brain and Learning*. Ed. Teyler. Stamford, Conn.: Greylock Publishers, 1978, pp. 138–145.

Helmut, Hirsch V. B., and D. N. Spinelli. "Modification of the Distribution of Receptive Field Orientation in Cats by Selective Visual Exposure During Development," *Exp. Brain Res.* Volume 13 (1971), pp. 509–527.

Kent, Saul. "Breaking the Age Barriers." *Health*, Volume 14: 6:24 (1982).

Peters, Michael N., M.D., and Charles T. Richardson, M.D. "Stressful Life Events, Acid Hypersecretion and Ulcer Disease." *Gastroenterology*, Volume 84–1 (January 1983), pp. 114–119.

"Science, Consciousness and Aging," *Proceedings of the International Conference*. Seelisberg, Switzerland: Maharishi European Research University, January 19–20, 1980.

Sheldrake, Rupert. "Hidden Force." *Science Digest,* Volume 89:9:54 (1981).

Simonton, Carl, M.D. *The Journal of Trans-Personal Psychology*, Volume 7, No. 1 (1975).

Stoler, Peter. "A Conversation with Jonas Salk." *Psychology Today*, Volume 17:3:50 (1983).

Vaillant, George E. "The Natural History of Male Psychologic Health." *New England Journal of Medicine*, Volume 301:23 (December 1979), pp. 1249–1254.

"The Vegetarian Approach to Eating." American Dietetic Association. Position paper No. 0000V. *Journal of the American Dietetic Association*, Volume 77 (July 1980): pp. 61–69.

Wallace, Robert Keith, Michael Dillbeck, Elijah Jacob, and Beth Harrington. *International Journal of Neuroscience,* Volume 16 (1982), pp. 53–58.

Weiner, Herbert, M.D., ed. "Stress and Ulcers—The Continuing Association." *Gastroenterology,* Volume 84–1 (January 1983), pp. 189–190.